Campath-1H

Emerging Frontline Therapy in Chronic Lymphocytic Leukemia

Campath-1H

Emerging Frontline Therapy in Chronic Lymphocytic Leukemia

Kanti R. Rai, MB, BS, FACP
Long Island Jewish Medical Center, New Hyde Park New York and Albert Einstein College of Medicine Bronx, New York, USA

and

Janet Stephenson, BSc (Hons), PhD
University of Leeds, CNAA, UK

The Parthenon Publishing Group
International Publishers in Medicine, Science & Technology

NEW YORK LONDON

Library of Congress Cataloging-in-Publication Data
Data available on application

British Library Cataloguing in Publication Data
Data available on application

Published in the USA by
The Parthenon Publishing Group Inc.
One Blue Hill Plaza
PO Box 1564, Pearl River
New York 10965, USA

Published in the UK and Europe by
The Parthenon Publishing Group Limited
Casterton Hall, Carnforth
Lancs, LA6 2LA, UK

ISBN 1-84214-060-4

Printed and bound by Butler & Tanner Ltd., Frome and London, UK

Contents

Foreword 7

Introduction 9

1
B-Cell Chronic Lymphocytic Leukemia:
Molecular Basis and Prognostic Markers 11

2
The Road to Remission: From Single Agent Intervention
to Combination Therapy and Onward 33

3
Monoclonal Antibodies in Cancer:
The Development of Campath-1H 51

4
Campath-1H in B-CLL:
Remission of Refractory Disease 71

5
The Role of Campath-1H Prior to BMT in Refractory B-CLL 87

Future Perspectives 111

Index 117

Foreword

Advances in monoclonal antibody use are likely to become the major theme in therapeutics during this first decade of the new millennium. Campath-1H stands alone among monoclonal antibodies because its reciprocal antigen CD52 is expressed on diverse cell types. Besides the already known role of Campath-1H in chronic lymphoproliferative disorders, its potential in the therapy of autoimmune diseases will be actively tested in the near future. It is quite likely, also, that the presence of CD52 in the epididymis, seminal fluid and spermatozoa will receive attention with respect to the future role of Campath-1H in yet another arena.

The purpose of this book is to provide a detailed overview of current knowledge of Campath-1H, and to present its further potential in clinical practise. We hope it will provide a balanced and informative text for the practitioner in hemato-oncology.

The authors wish to dedicate this volume to Herman Waldmann and Geoffrey Hale, both of whom were kind enough to read and comment upon the proofs. These pioneers took Campath-1H from its initial discovery through various developmental stages to clinical application, and we are most grateful for their guidance and expertise.

Kanti R. Rai and Janet Stephenson

Introduction

The story of the development of the monoclonal antibody Campath-1H is a fascinating one. This history is all the more relevant today as clinical trials demonstrate that Campath-1H is an effective salvage treatment for B-cell chronic lymphocytic leukemia.

B-CLL, in past decades, has consistently defied attempts at a permanent purge and/or curative bone marrow transplant. Worse, relapsed disease after chemotherapy is almost invariably refractory to re-treatment with the same drugs. The prolonged clinical course of B-CLL has meant that, until now, treatment has been palliative and undertaken only when the patient showed signs of advancing disease. This traditional approach is now beginning to change in the light of new developments that offer the promise of curbing progressive disease. The successful induction of programmed cell death by nucleoside analogues, large-scale purging of B-cells using Campath-1H, and advances in stem cell transplantation have all contributed towards a new goal: preventing progression and eradicating residual disease.

Campath-1H therapy targets CD52, found on normal, mature lymphocytes as well as their malignant counterparts. In B-CLL, Campath-1H is particularly effective in clearing lymphocytes from blood and bone marrow, with significant clinical benefit. Peripheral blood stem cells can be successfully mobilized and harvested from Campath-1H-treated patients, therefore the opportunity for autologous stem cell transplantation is maintained for these patients. In addition, the ability to control graft-versus-host (GVHD) disease by depleting donor and host T-cells, gives Campath-1H a role in non-myeloablative conditioning prior to allogeneic stem cell transplantation.

Campath-1H therapy has induced remission in a number of previously heavily-treated, poor-prognosis, fludarabine-refractory B-CLL patients, and several ongoing clinical trials only hint at future achievements that may build on this promising beginning. The task at hand is to fulfill this promise of Campath-1H, perhaps in combination with fludarabine, for as many patients with refractory B-CLL as possible. Perhaps long-term control of this disease is possible now and patients may finally achieve lasting and complete remissions.

For those patients with previously untreated B-CLL, Campath-1H perhaps heralds a new era in management and outcome. The eradication of malignant clones from blood and bone marrow suggests that Campath-1H in conjunction with emerging prognostic markers will see early treatment for this patient group. Furthermore, since this treatment is no barrier to autologous stem cell transplantation and reduces the risk of GVHD for allografting, it seems probable that future algorithms will incorporate Campath-1H for treatment-naïve patients.

This volume records the development and actions of Campath-1H, presents the unique clinical, immunological and molecular features of B-CLL, and explores the potential of Campath-1H as frontline therapy for patients with B-CLL.

1

B-Cell Chronic Lymphocytic Leukemia: Molecular Basis and Prognostic Markers

B-cell chronic lymphocytic leukemia (B-CLL) is a slow, prevalent killer, the most common form of leukemia in the Western world. It accounts for approximately 9% of all cancers and 30% of all leukemias[1], with 12,000 new cases being diagnosed each year in the United States alone[2], and two-thirds of these new cases being patients over 60 years of age.

Diagnosis is based on criteria established by the International Workshop on CLL (IWCLL) and the National Cancer Institute Workshop (NCIW). These include a sustained lymphocytosis, a bone marrow aspirate of greater than 30% lymphocytes and the presence of neoplastic cells of B-cell origin which express the B-cell markers, CD19, CD20 and CD23 in addition to the T-cell marker CD5. They also show weak expression of surface immunoglobulin.

Assessment of disease severity is usually based on the Binet staging system in Europe[3] or the Rai staging system[4] in the USA (Tables 1 and 2). Disease is graded according to the extent of lymphocytosis, enlargement of lymph nodes, liver and spleen and the degree of impairment of normal hematopoiesis.

Table 1. Rai staging system for B-CLL

Risk	Rai stage	5-year survival	Clinical features
Low	0	approx 98%	Lymphocytosis in blood and bone marrow only
Intermediate	I	approx 95%	Lymphocytosis and lymphadenopathy
	II	approx 88%	Lymphocytosis plus hepatomegaly or splenomegaly or both
High	III	< 5%	Lymphocytosis and anemia
	IV	0%	Lymphocytosis and thrombocytopenia

Table 2. Binet staging system for B-CLL

Binet stage	5-year survival	Hemoglobin and platelet counts	Clinical features
A	approx 90%	Hemoglobin > 10 g/dl Platelets > 100 x 10^9/l	< 2 node-bearing or enlarged areas*
B	approx 63%	Hemoglobin > 10 g/dl Platelets > 100 x 10^9/l	> 3 node-bearing or enlarged areas
C	approx 40%	Hemoglobin < 10 g/dl and/or Platelets < 100 x 10^9/l	Any number of node-bearing or enlarged areas

*Cervical, axillary, inguinal (unilateral or bilateral), spleen and liver each count as one area

B-CLL also exhibits a high frequency of auto-immune phenomena[5] causing it to be described as a malignancy of anti-self B-cells[6]. Monoclonal polyreactive IgM antibodies, able to bind two or more antigens, although often with low affinity, are detectable on the cell surface and in the serum of patients with the disease[7–9]. In addition to this self-reactive phenomenon, patients generally acquire an immunodeficiency characterized by hypogammaglobulinemia, impaired production of secondary immunoglobulin isotypes, diminished germinal center formation and increased susceptibility to bacterial infections. Prior to treatment the most common pathogens are those which require opsonization for bacterial killing, such as *Staphylococcus* spp., *Streptococcus pneumoniae* and *Haemophilus influenzae*, while after treatment there are more infections with Gram-negative and opportunistic organisms[10].

Chromosomal abnormalities are frequent in B-CLL cells (reviewed in Juliusson and Merup, 1998[11]. While initially abnormalities were estimated to be present in approximately 50% of cases, studies have been hampered by the difficulty of getting B-CLL cells, which are predominantly in the resting phase of the cell cycle, to undergo mitosis. Two advances are currently revealing the true incidence. These are the advent of sensitive detection methods such as fluorescent *in situ* hybridization (FISH), which can be used to detect changes during interphase, and optimization of mitosis-induction protocols for B-CLL cells.

Such protocols now allow 90% of cases to be informative[12,13]. Conventional cytogenetics remain important to detect complex karyotypes, which are associated with a poor prognosis. Studies using FISH show chromosomal abnormalities occurring in up to 70% of patients, the most common being trisomy 12, and deletions or translocations of chromosome 13q14[11,14,15]. Some abnormalities are associated with distinctive phenotypes (Table 3). Deletions of 11q23.1 are seen in B-CLL cells with a greatly reduced ability to produce a number of cell adhesion molecules such as integrins, CD48 and CD58α. These patients have extensive lymphadenopathy, infiltrative disease and short survival times. Deletions of 17p that remove the tumor suppressor gene p53 are associated with the rapid development of resistance to chemotherapy and progressive disease, and are an independent marker for poor survival. Deletions of 6q and of 13q14.1, when they are the sole chromosomal abnormality, are indicators of benign disease.

Table 3. Chromosomal abnormalities in B-CLL

Abnormality	Frequency	Candidate gene	Prognostic significance	Ref
Complex karyotype	approx 5%		Progressive disease	13
Trisomy 12	approx 22–34%	?	Progressive disease	11,16,17
del 13q14.3	approx 40%	Leu 6	Benign disease	11,18–20
del 11q23.1	approx 5–15%	Adhesion molecules	Bone marrow infiltration, progressive disease	15,21
del 17p	approx 10%	p53 (confirmed)	Chemoresistance, progressive disease	22
del 6q	approx 7%	TNF-α?	Larger tumor mass no inferior outcome unless del 6q is secondary to trisomy-12	23,24
t(11;14) (q13;q32)	2–5%	?	CLL/PL, transformation into PLL, overlap with mantle cell leukemia	25

Epidemiological studies over a number of years have shown an elevated familial risk for CLL, more so than for any other form of leukemia[26,27]. Many of the families show vertical transmission consistent with the expression of an autosomal dominant trait. As demonstrated using the Utah population database, individuals within such families are three to six times more likely to develop CLL than the general population[28–30]. Unlike acute leukemia and chronic granulocytic leukemia, CLL has not been associated with prior irradiation. In addition, the low incidence of the disease among certain ethnic groups, such as Asians who continue to show low levels even after migration to USA[31], suggests that genetic factors are stronger than environmental factors. Another feature of familial CLL is anticipation, in which the disorder shows increased severity and earlier age of onset in each generation[32].

The natural clinical course of the disease is highly variable. In patients with disease defined as early, and with no additional prognostic indicators such as underlying cytogenetic abnormalities, life expectancy is almost unaltered compared with normal controls. However, patients with advanced CLL usually face a progressive disorder with a median survival of less than two years.

This pattern, of a long plateau followed by a rapid downhill slide, renders one question of prime importance: when to treat the disease? Too early, and the patient will reap no benefits, while still undergoing the rigors of chemotherapy, and very possibly will develop secondary malignancies as a consequence of treatment. Too late, and the prognosis is grim; since the extent of the disease at diagnosis is the main determinant of final outcome.

As yet, the molecular basis for the changes which occur when a patient moves into the final stages of the disease has not been well-defined. The last few years have, however, seen a great deal of progress in elucidating the nature of the aberrant B-cell and the features relevant to therapeutic intervention.

The abnormal cell in B-CLL

At the cellular/molecular level, CLL is a disease of abnormal cell death regulation rather than increased proliferation. The aberrant B-cells accumulate slowly but inexorably. Key features show them to be:

- mature CD5+ B-cells
- slow to divide
- protected from programmed cell death

The B-CLL CD5+ cell and its normal counterpart

B-CLL cells are regarded as CD5+ if greater than 95% express this marker, highly expressed on normal T-cells, with 93% of cases of CLL being CD5+[33]. The small proportion of B-cell leukemias that do not express CD5 are either not classifiable as chronic lymphocytic leukemia[34] or can be assessed as a subset of the disease[35].

Normal CD5+ B-cells (B1 cells) arise early in ontogeny. Present throughout fetal tissue, in the adult they are restricted to the peritoneal cavity and to the mantle zone of lymph nodes[36].

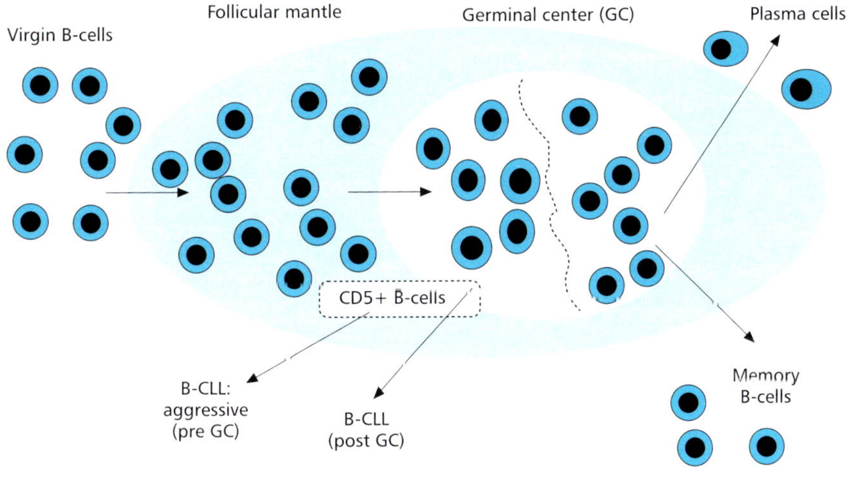

Figure 1. B-cell differentiation in B-CLL

Mature B-cells undergo a further process of differentiation within the secondary follicle (Figure 1). Beginning as virgin cells, they pass into the follicular mantle (pre-germinal center, GC) then pass into the GC, progressing from centroblasts to centrocytes and finally developing into plasma cells and memory B-cells (post GC)[37]. Virgin cells have already undergone the germline rearrangements which shuffle IgG coding sequences to generate immune diversity. During transit through the germinal center, B-cells then acquire additional IgG variability by point mutations in hypermutable regions of variable (V) sequences. Analysis of the presence or absence of such somatic point mutation in chronic lymphocytic leukemia has shown that they occur in about 25% to 50% B-CLL cases[38], indicating which CD5+ leukemic cells have passed through the germinal center, and so may be regarded as possessing some of the activated characteristics of memory B-cells. Furthermore, unmutated V sequences are found in the more aggressive forms of the disease[39–41]. This leads to the conclusion that there are two forms of B-CLL; a more benign form arising from a cell which has passed through the germinal center, and a more aggressive form arising from a naïve B-cell. The presence or absence of such mutation is increasingly being used as a powerful prognostic marker since unmutated V sequences define a subgroup of patients (approximately 40%) with increased risk of disease progression.

In addition, where virgin B-cells produce IgG using all possible variable (V) sequences, the CD5+ subpopulation exhibits a restricted antibody repertoire[42], with a bias towards the production of polyreactive low-affinity autoantibodies, antibodies capable of recognizing multiple structurally dissimilar antigens[43]. The autoreactive component is an acknowledged component of the normal B-cell repertoire. Normal auto-reactive antibodies (NAA) bind public epitopes expressed by all individuals in a species and even across species. Their low affinity and broad specificity allows them to bind self- and non-self antigens such as microbial antigens. Originally NAA are thought to have evolved in animals with no ability to make highly-specific high-affinity antibodies and in humans they now perform as a first-line defense against infection, during the window required for the initiation and amplification of specific immune responses.

CD5+ B1 cells are a self-replenishing lymphocyte population and have been shown to constitutively express STAT3, a signal transducer and activator of transcription implicated in the process of self-renewal[44,45]. They are also unusual in expressing the protein kinase Lck which has a crucial role in T-cell activation[46].

The abnormal B-CLL cell population shares these self-renewal abilities and the production of polyreactive autoantibodies with consequent ability to form rosettes with mouse erythrocytes *in vitro* (Figure 2).

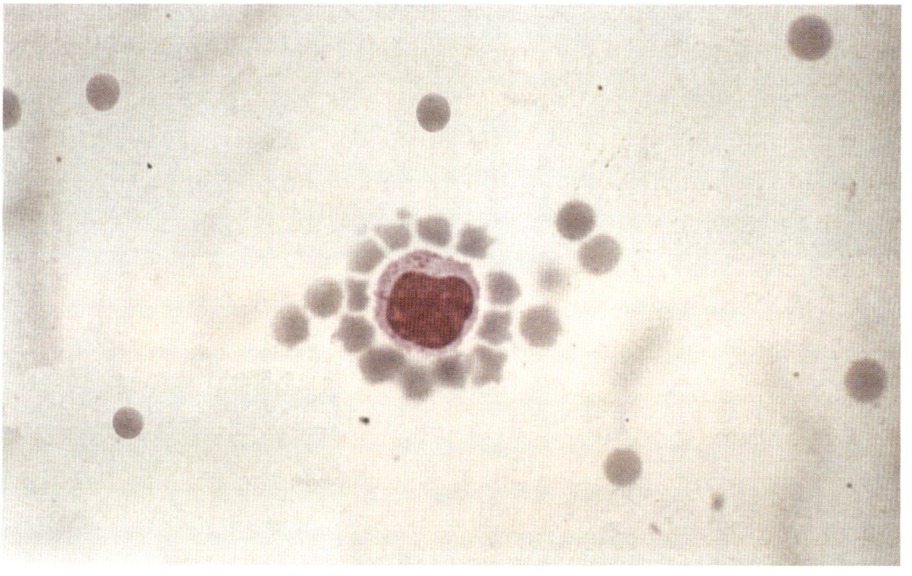

Figure 2. Rosette formation by B-CLL lymphocytes

The pathogenic auto-antibodies detectable in up to 30% of patients are usually polyclonal and directed against hematopoietic antigens expressed on the surface of red blood cells, and, more rarely, on the surface of platelets[47–49]. These may lead to severe autoimmune hemolytic anemia and/or thrombocytopenia[50]. While auto-immune thrombocytopenia is seen in only 2% of cases, a larger proportion of patients have an increase in platelet-associated IgGs[51]. The basis for such auto-immune phenomena in B-CLL and the high (up to 60%) incidence of hypogammaglobulinemia leading to infectious complications such as *Streptococcus pneumoniae* infection is poorly understood.

The potential role of T-cell defects in inducing auto-immune complications in B-CLL has been stressed by recent data showing an increase in auto-immune hemolytic anemia after treatment with drugs such as purine analogues which deplete CD4[52] and, to a lesser extent, CD8 T-cell counts[53]. Other work showing the influence of T-cells on the malignant clone have demonstrated a striking redistribution of

CD4+ helper cells into involved bone marrow and lymph nodes[54]. These cells are oligoclonal and the extent of their expansion is a measure of disease duration.

The sites where B-CLL cells are induced to proliferate are not fully established but the best candidates are the pseudo-follicles (or proliferation centers) apparent in 90% of cases. These resemble normal secondary lymphoid follicles in that they consist of B-CLL and T-cells in a delicate network of follicular dendritic cells, although, unlike a normal secondary follicle, the numbers of B-cells predominate. The abnormal cell in B-CLL corresponds, in some of its characteristics, more closely to recirculating follicular cells than to classic B1 cells. These follicular cells have migrated into the T-cell-rich areas of secondary lymphoid tissues and the red pulp of the spleen where they have been primed, an intervention which involves protection from apoptotic cell death, to recirculate between the follicles of secondary lymphoid tissue.

The surface membrane phenotype of the malignant cells in B-CLL is shown in Table 4.

Table 4. Surface membrane phenotype of malignant B-CLL B-cells

	Augmented or normal level of expression		Decreased level of expression
	Membrane	**Soluble**	
Lineage markers	CD5, CD19, CD20, CD21, CD22, CD24	CD22	IgM/IgD, CD10
Cytokine receptors	CD25, CD119, CD124, IL-4, IL-6, TNF		
B-cell/T-cell coreceptors	CD40, CD72	CD40	MHC Class I, Class II, CD80
Integrins	CD54, CD11a, CD18, CD58		
Other	CD23, CD43, CD95, CD36, CD38, CD44	β2-microglobulin	CD45, CD71

The CD5+ cells in B-CLL express a number of cell surface markers not found on their normal B1 or recirculating counterpart. These include the thrombospondin receptor, CD36[55], correlated with diffuse bone marrow histology, and likely to be involved in tumor spreading, dipeptidylpeptidase IV, CD26, recently identified as a marker of B-CLL[56], CD38, which identifies a subset of B-CLL cells not susceptible to induction of apoptosis[57,58], and CD44, associated with aggressive disease[59,60].

Normal CD5+ cell phenotype is synchronized to cell cycle stage. B-CLL cells differ, possessing an ability to show phenotypic activation and express several B-cell activation-associated antigens, while still remaining in what has historically been considered as a fully resting stage of the cell cycle. Now, investigation of B-CLL cells and the balance sustained between proliferation and survival enhancement are offering new insights into G_0 and the G_0/G_1 boundary of the cell cycle.

Slow proliferators

B-CLL cells have a relatively long lifespan, and though they divide so seldom, the population of such cells gradually expands until it dominates over a population of normal cells. The leukemic cells in CLL are maintained in the G_0 phase of the cell cycle, and respond more weakly to mitogenic signals than normal B-cells, as shown in Figure 3.

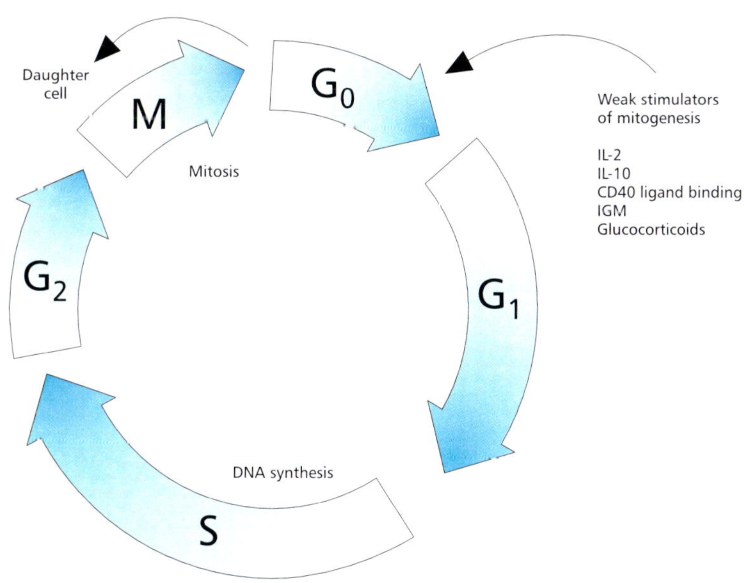

Figure 3. Cell cycle signalling in B-CLL

Investigation of weak proliferation in B-CLL has focused on the B-cell antigen receptor complex (BCR)[61] which is a multimeric complex formed by the surface immunoglobulin (sIg) homodimer and the noncovalently bound heterodimer CD79a/CD79b, (α and β immunoglobulin chains) in association with other cell surface antigens, including CD5, CD19, CD21, CD22, and CD81. Triggering of the receptor complex would normally activate protein tyrosine kinases and induce mobilization of intracellular Ca^{2+}, but signal transduction in the B-CLL cell appears to be blocked. Defective CD79a, the Ig α chain, may be responsible for this, since it has been found to be altered by point mutation, deletion and insertion in the majority of B-CLL clones[62–64]. Heterodimer integrity is essential for Ig to reach the membrane, for initiation of signal transduction, to correct antigen presentation and for mediation of BCR-induced apoptosis[65]. Other membrane molecules such as the CD19/CD21 complex and CD22 have roles as accessories in B-cell signal transduction. The CD19/CD21 complex serves as a general regulator of B-cell response, while the stimulation of CD22 potentiates the proliferation induced by anti-IgG.

Protection from programmed cell death

BCL-2

B-CLL is the archetypal example of a disorder caused by a failure in programmed cell death (PCD) or apoptosis. The anti-apoptotic protein BCL-2 is overexpressed in most B-CLL cases, although, unlike follicular non-Hodgkin's lymphoma, this overexpression is not accompanied by a t(14;18) chromosomal translocation.

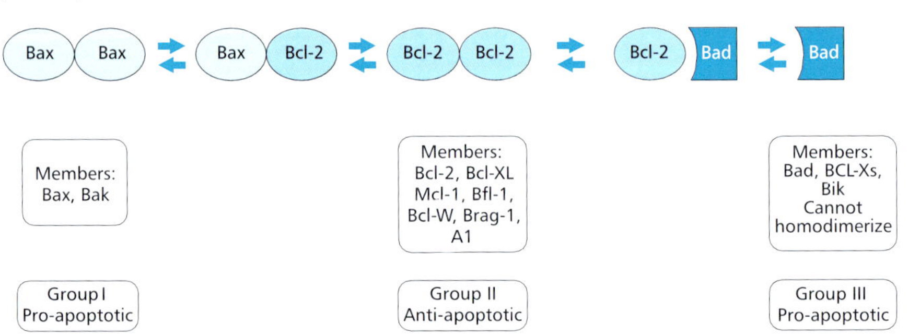

Figure 4. BCL-2 family proteins

In vitro overexpression of BCL-2 can block or impair the initiation of apoptosis by every known anti-cancer drug, including purine nucleosides[66,67].

Expression of BCL-2 and homologues, BCL-XL, MCL-1, BFL-1, and BCL-W, or antagonists, BAX, and BAK, (see Figure 4), could be a major influence on chemosensitivity. A high Bcl/Bax protein ratio is frequently seen in patients found to be clinically unresponsive to therapy[68].

However, because overexpression of BCL-2 is so widespread in B-CLL, examination of relative levels has not been particularly helpful in predicting clinical outcome[69]. Nor, because of the need to investigate the entire extended Bcl-2 protein family, has limited *in vitro* sensitivity data proved to be useful in predicting response[70].

One anti-cancer strategy has pursued the use of anti-sense oligonucleotides; short sequences of synthetic nucleic acids complementary to the BCL-2 mRNA, in order to down-modulate Bcl-2 expression. Such treatment is aimed at overcoming resistance to chemotherapy using apoptosis-inducing agents, and has shown some benefits in non-Hodgkin's lymphoma[71].

Protection from apoptosis is an active process, sustained by continual external stimulation. B-CLL lymphocytes grown in culture in the absence of growth factors will spontaneously decrease production of Bcl-2 and undergo apoptosis. *In vitro* studies have allowed some of the molecular mechanisms behind the increase in the Bcl-2/Bax ratio to be defined, with growth factors assigned a role in apoptotic cell death.

Table 5. Growth factor stimuli in B-CLL

Group I – BCL 2 expression **enhanced**, apoptosis **decreased**	**Refs**	Group II – BCL-2 expression **reduced**, apoptosis **increased**	**Refs**
IL-4*	72–75	IgM	83
IL-6	73	Glucocorticoids	84
IL-8	76	IL-10	73,85,86
bFGF	77	IL-15	87
Thioredoxin	78		
CD6 activation	79		
CD40 activation	80		
TNF-α	81		
IFN-γ	72,82		
IFN-α → STAT3	72		

*Note: IL-4 highly dependent on presence of co-stimulators for anti-apoptotic effect

Some of the stimuli included in Group I, Table 5, are synergistic in their effects. Thioredoxin (Trx) is a potent costimulator with IL-1 and TNF-α and stimulates autocrine TNF-α release, further protecting against apoptotic cell death.

Results of *in vitro* studies on the effects of modulators on proliferation and apoptosis support the use of IL-10[73,86] for immune therapy of early B-CLL and IFN-γ[82] for therapy of the disease in the later stages.

This current emphasis on the effects of input from external signals, and the large number of such stimuli able to rescue the B-cell from cell death, directs attention in the analysis and treatment of B-CLL towards B-cell cross-talk with cells from other lineages. These include bone marrow fibroblasts and stromal cells[88], antigen-presenting follicular dendritic cells, and, most importantly, T-cells.

While the Bcl-2/Bax ratio within the cell is controlled by stimulation of some cell surface proteins by cytokines and glucocorticoids, other cell surface receptors act via cytoplasmic molecules other than Bcl-2. These include both Fas (CD95) and CD40 and other members of the tumor necrosis factor receptor superfamily. CD40 acts via NFκβ, and Fas acts directly via cascades of caspases, ultimately promoting DNA fragmentation, as shown in Figure 5.

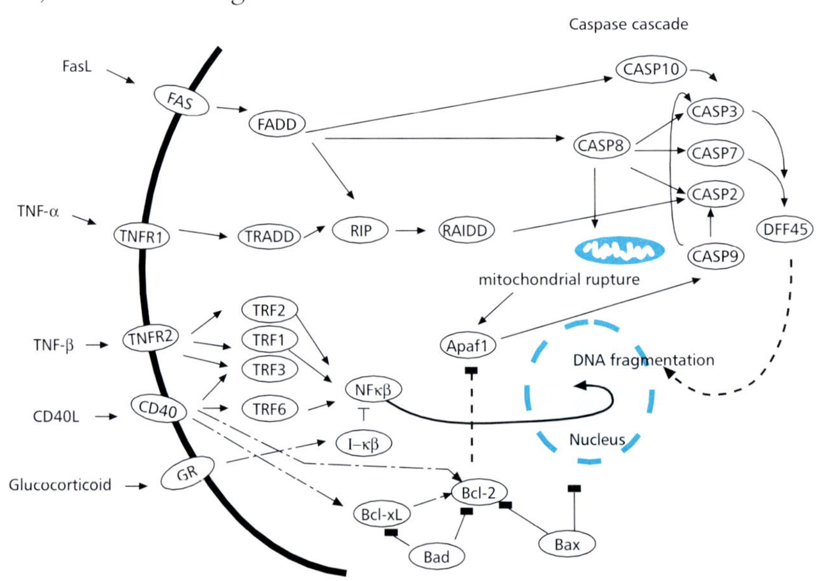

Figure 5. Pathways to apoptosis

Caspases are present in all cells as inactive proteins and are activated by proteolytic cleavage into two subunits in response to apoptotic stimulation.

B-CLL cells may have developed additional molecular mechanisms to circumvent apoptosis via these pathways, normally triggered by molecules such as Fas.

Fas

Fas (CD95) is normally expressed by germinal center and memory B-cells, and its ligand FasL is found on activated T-cells and natural killer (NK) cells. The Fas/FasLigand system is ordinarily responsible for clonal deletion of autoreactive T-cells, and cytotoxic T-cell (CTC)-mediated cell lysis. Acquisition of defects in these molecules is associated with lymphoproliferation and autoimmunity.

B-CLL cells are negative or weakly positive for Fas expression. Although they can be induced to express Fas, they remain resistant to Fas-mediated apoptosis. While mutations in FASL have been associated with resistance to apoptosis in inherited autoimmune proliferative syndromes[89], sequencing FAS or FASL DNA from B-CLL patients has not found mutation[90]. Cytoplasmic molecules have been identified which are capable of blocking apoptosis in response to Fas[91]. These have not, as yet, been studied widely in CLL, although Fas-resistance after stimulus of B-CLL cells in culture with CD40L is accompanied by increased expression of the Fas antagonist, FLIP[92].

Activated B-CLL cells have been found to release soluble forms of Fas and FasL[93] and *in vitro* studies[83,94] have found constitutive expression of Fas and FasL. While the role of Fas/FasL interactions in B-CLL is still unclear, such work has raised the possibility that early CLL cells are apoptosis defective because they fail to express Fas, while in later stages, progressive cells express cell surface and soluble forms of both Fas and FasL. According to this model, the soluble form of Fas competes for CTC cells bearing FasL, reducing interaction at the cell surface, and the soluble form of FasL binds to CTC cells mediating T-cell death, so not only resisting apoptosis but also constituting a mechanism to evade the immune response.

Soluble proteins as markers of disease

Progression in B-CLL is accompanied by the detection of increasing amounts of soluble forms of other proteins, released from their normal sites on the cell membrane by proteolytic cleavage, and a number of these are useful as prognostic markers.

Serum levels of IL-8, a cytokine able to inhibit apoptosis via FAS and BCL-2, correlate with intracellular levels of BCL-2 and may be useful as a marker of the pace of progression in intermediate disease[76]. The adhesion molecule CD44, a proteoglycan which participates in a variety of functions, including lymphohematopoiesis, lymphocyte homing and tumor metastasis, is also found in the serum as a marker of disease progression in both non-Hodgkin's lymphoma and B-CLL[95]. Soluble CD21 is also found in B-CLL[96] where it interferes with T-cell-dependent immunoregulation.

Soluble CD27[97], β2-microglobulin and IL2R can be used as markers of total tumor mass (TTM), while sCD14 is correlated with IgG serum values and the soluble form of the adhesion molecule ICAM-1 is correlated to the ability of tumor to spread[98]. Serum CD23 concentration is a reliable disease marker of both lymphocytosis and TTM[99,100].

Serum CD23 levels have also been assessed for prognostic value in patients with early disease, most recently in work by Desablens[101] in which the majority of 156 patients were in Binet stage A (131 patients). At a median follow-up of 7.5 years, analysis of factors associated with progression has allowed cut-off points for serum CD23 and β2-microglobulin to be set (33 U, and 3 mg, respectively). Stratification using these cut-off points in combination predicts survival better than using Binet staging.

The identification of such reliable markers of tumor mass and of disease progression is now being used in newly initiated clinical trials in which assessment of tumor mass, in addition to assessment by Rai or Binet criteria alone, is used to facilitate the decision of whether to treat or not to treat the disease[102]. The Rai and Binet staging systems have some disadvantages, particularly in the design of clinical trials, since while they are simple, effective and unbiased staging systems, they are not ideal for assessment of the dynamics of the disease, since the advanced stages of

B-CLL are defined by bone marrow failure irrespective of tumor load. Assessment of tumor mass is becoming increasingly important to supplement other staging criteria and also to aid assessment of response to treatment.

Summary

Work on the unique clinical, immunological and molecular features of B-CLL has defined a number of aspects associated with progression of the disease. Aggressive disease is correlated with:

- trisomy 12
- unmutated immunoglobulin genes (pre-germinal center)
- solubilized cell surface markers
- high serum β2-microglobulin

Protocols for disease treatment are increasingly being devised to take advantage of significant aspects of B-CLL cell metabolism, such as apoptosis-induction by a variety of methods, amongst which is the highly successful intervention with the nucleoside analogue fludarabine phosphate. Effective markers for disease progression will also facilitate the decision of when to intervene in the course of the disease.

Other characteristics of B-CLL, such as the molecular cross-talk which occurs between B- and T-cells, and ways by which these malignant cells evade the immune system, require further, focused research for clearer insight into these aspects of the disease.

Reference List

1. Kipps TJ. Chronic lymphocytic leukemia and related diseases. *Williams Hematology*. New York: McGraw-Hill; 1995:1017–1324

2. Wingo PA, Tong T, Bolden S. Cancer statistics, 1995. *CA Cancer J Clin*. 1995;45:8–30

3. Binet JL, Auquier A, Dighiero G, Chastang C, Piguet H, Goasguen J, Vaugier G, Potron G, Colona P, Oberling F, Thomas M, Tchernia G, Jacquillat C, Boivin P, Lesty C, Duault MT, Monconduit M, Belabbes S, Gremy F. A new prognostic classification of chronic lymphocytic leukemia derived from a multivariate survival analysis. *Cancer*. 1981;48:198–206

4. Rai KR, Sawitsky A, Cronkite EP, Chanana AD, Levy RN, Pasternack BS. Clinical staging of chronic lymphocytic leukemia. *Blood*. 1975;46:219–234

5. Kipps TJ. Immunoglobulin genes in chronic lymphocytic leukemia. *Blood Cells*. 1993;19: 615–612

6. Caligaris-Cappio F. B-Chronic lymphocytic leukemia: a malignancy of anti-self in B-cells. *Blood*. 1996;87:2615–2620

7. Preud'Homme JL, Seligmann, M. Anti-human immunoglobulin G activity of membrane bound immunoglobulin M in lymphoproliferative disorders. *Proc Natl Acad Sci USA*. 1978; 69:2132–2138

8. Borche L, Lim A, Binet JL, Dighiero G. Evidence that chronic lymphocytic leukemia B lymphocytes are frequently committed to production of natural autoantibodies. *Blood*. 1990;76:562–569

9. Kipps TJ, Robbins BA, Kuster P, Carson DA. Autoantibody-associated cross-reactive idiotypes expressed at high frequency in chronic lymphocytic leukemia relative to B-cell lymphomas of follicular center cell origin. *Blood*. 1988;72:422–428

10. Kalil N, Cheson BD. Management of chronic lymphocytic leukaemia. *Drugs Aging*. 2000; 16:9–27

11. Juliusson G, Merup M. Cytogenetics in chronic lymphocytic leukemia. *Semin Oncol*. 1998; 25:19–25

12. Larramendy ML, Siitonen SM, Zhu Y, Hurme M, Vilpo L, Vilpo JA, Knuutila S. Optimized mitogen stimulation induces proliferation of neoplastic B cells in chronic lymphocytic leukemia: significance for cytogenetic analysis.The Tampere Chronic Lympocytic Leukemia group. *Cytogenet Cell Genet*. 1998;82:215–221

13. Geisler CH, Philip P, Christensen BE, Hou-Jensen K, Pedersen NT, Jensen OM, Thorling K, Andersen E, Birgens HS, Drivsholm A, Ellegaard J, Larsen JK, Plesner T, Brown P, Andersen PK, Hansen MM. In B-cell chronic lymphocytic leukaemia chromosome 17 abnormalities and not trisomy 12 are the single most important cytogenetic abnormalities for the prognosis: a cytogenetic and immunophenotypic study of 480 unselected newly diagnosed patients. *Leuk Res*. 1997;21:1011–1023

14. Dohner H, Stilgenbauer S, Benner A, Leupolt E, Krober A, Bullinger L, Dohner K, Bentz M, Lichter P. Genomic aberrations and survival in chronic lymphocytic leukemia. *N Engl J Med*. 2000;343:1910–1916

15. Zhu Y, Monni O, El-Rifai W, Siitonen SM, Vilpo L, Vilpo J, Knuutila S. Discontinuous deletions at 11q23 in B cell chronic lymphocytic leukemia. *Leukemia*. 1999;13:708–712

16. Caligaris-Cappio F, Hamblin TJ. B-cell chronic lymphocytic leukemia: a bird of a different feather. *J Clin Oncol*. 1999;17:399–408

17. Liso V, Capalbo S, Lapietra A, Pavone V, Guarini A, Specchia G. Evaluation of trisomy 12 by fluorescence in situ hybridization in peripheral blood, bone marrow and lymph nodes of patients with B-cell chronic lymphocytic leukemia. *Haematologica*. 1999;84:212–217

18. Hogan WJ, Tefferi A, Borell TJ, Jenkins R, Li CY, Witzig TE. Prognostic relevance of monosomy at the 13q14 locus detected by fluorescence in situ hybridization in B-cell chronic lymphocytic leukemia. *Cancer Genet Cytogenet.* 1999;110:77–81

19. Corcoran MM, Rasool O, Liu Y, Iyengar A, Grander D, Ibbotson RE, Merup M, Wu X, Brodyansky V, Gardiner AC, Juliusson G, Chapman RM, Ivanova G, Tiller M, Gahrton G, Yankovsky N, Zabarovsky E, Oscier DG, Einhorn S. Detailed molecular delineation of 13q14.3 loss in B-cell chronic lymphocytic leukemia. *Blood.* 1998;91:1382–1390

20. Rondeau G, Moreau I, Bezieau S, Cadoret E, Moisan JP, Devilder MC. Exclusion of Leu1 and Leu2 genes as tumor suppressor genes in 13q14.3-deleted B-CLL. *Leukemia.* 1999;13: 1630–1632

21. Sembries S, Pahl H, Stilgenbauer S, Dohner H, Schriever F. Reduced expression of adhesion molecules and cell signaling receptors by chronic lymphocytic leukemia cells with 11q deletion. *Blood.* 1999;93:624–631

22. Dohner H, Stilgenbauer S, Dohner K, Bentz M, Lichter P. Chromosome aberrations in B-cell chronic lymphocytic leukemia: reassessment based on molecular cytogenetic analysis. *J Mol Med.* 1999;77:266–281

23. Finn WG, Kay NE, Kroft SH, Church S, Peterson LC. Secondary abnormalities of chromosome 6q in B-cell chronic lymphocytic leukemia: a sequential study of karyotypic instability in 51 patients. *Am J Hematol.* 1998;59:223–229

24. Stilgenbauer S, Dohner K, Bentz M, Lichter P, Dohner H. Molecular cytogenetic analysis of B-cell chronic lymphocytic leukemia. *Ann Hematol.* 1998;76:101–110

25. Dierlamm J, Michaux, L, Criel, A, Wloddarska, I, Van den Berghe, H, Hossfeld, DK. Genetic abnormalities in chronic lymphocytic leukemia and their clinical and prognostic implications. *Cancer Genet Cytogenet.* 1997;94:27–34

26. Linet MS, Blattner WA. The epidemiology of chronic lymphocytic leukemia. In: Pollack A, Catovsky D, eds. *Chronic Lymphocytic Leukemia*. Chu, Switzerland: Harwood; 1988:11

27. Linet MS, Van Natta ML, Brookmeyer R, Khoury MJ, McCaffrey LD, Humphrey RL, Szklo M. Familial cancer history and chronic lymphocytic leukemia. A case-control study. *Am J Epidemiol.* 1989;130:655–664

28. Goldgar DE, Easton DF, Cannon-Albright LA, Skolnick MH. Systematic population-based assessment of cancer risk in first-degree relatives of cancer probands. *J Natl Cancer Inst.* 1994;86:1600–1608

29. Cannon-Albright LA, Thomas A, Goldgar DE, Gholami K, Rowe K, Jacobsen M, McWhorter WP, Skolnick MH. Familiality of cancer in Utah. *Cancer Res.* 1994;54:2378–2385

30. Gunz FW, Gunz JP, Veale AM, Chapman CJ, Houston IB. Familial leukaemia: a study of 909 families. *Scand J Haematol.* 1975;15:117–131

31. Gale RP, Cozen W, Goodman MT, Wang FF, Bernstein L. Decreased chronic lymphocytic leukemia incidence in Asians in Los Angeles County. *Leuk Res.* 2000;24:665–669

32. Horwitz M, Goode EL, Jarvik GP. Anticipation in familial leukemia. *Am J Hum Genet.* 1996; 59:990–998

33. Cartron G, Linassier C, Bremond JL, Desablens B, Georget MT, Fimbel B, Luthier F, Dutel JL, Lamagnere JP, Colombat P. CD5 negative B-cell chronic lymphocytic leukemia: clinical and biological features of 42 cases. *Leuk Lymphoma.* 1998;31:209–216

34. Huang JC, Finn WG, Goolsby CL, Variakojis D, Peterson LC. CD5- small B-cell leukemias are rarely classifiable as chronic lymphocytic leukemia. *Am J Clin Pathol.* 1999;111:123–130

35. Pangalis GA, Angelopoulou MK, Vassilakopoulos TP, Siakantaris MP, Kittas C. B-chronic lymphocytic leukemia, small lymphocytic lymphoma, and lymphoplasmacytic lymphoma, including Waldenström's macroglobulinemia: a clinical, morphologic, and biologic spectrum of similar disorders. *Semin Hematol.* 1999;36:104–114

36. Kantor AB. The development and repertoire of B-1 cells (CD5 B cells). *Immunol Today.* 1991;12:389–391

37. Gaidano G, Carbone, A. Mum1: A step ahead toward the understanding of lymphoma biogenesis. *Leukemia.* 2000;14:563–566

38. Mavridis AK, Tsiara S, Makis A, Chaidos A, Christou L, Seferiadis K, Bourantas KL. Interleukins, TNF-alpha and beta-2M in patients with B cell chronic lymphocytic leukemia. *J Exp Clin Cancer Res.* 1998;17:445–448

39. Damle RN, Wasil T, Fais F, Ghiotto F, Valetto A, Allen SL, Buchbinder A, Budman D, Dittmar K, Kolitz J, Lichtman SM, Schulman P, Vinciguerra VP, Rai KR, Ferrarini M, Chiorazzi N. Ig V gene mutation status and CD38 expression as novel prognostic indicators in chronic lymphocytic leukemia. *Blood.* 1999;94:1840–1847

40. Hamblin TJ, Davis Z, Gardiner A, Oscier DG, Stevenson FK. Unmutated Ig V(H) genes are associated with a more aggressive form of chronic lymphocytic leukemia. *Blood.* 1999; 94:1848–1854

41. Soderberg O. Growth and survival of B-chronic lymphocytic leukaemia cells. *Med Oncol.* 1998;15:73-78

42. Kantor AB, Herzenberg LA. Origin of murine B cell lineages. *Annu Rev Immunol.* 1993; 11:501–538

43. Ramsland PA, Brock CR, Moses J, Robinson BG, Edmundson AB, Raison RL. Structural aspects of human IgM antibodies expressed in chronic B lymphocytic leukemia. *Immunotechnology.* 1999;4:217–229

44. Karras JG, Wang Z, Huo L, Howard RG, Frank DA, Rothstein TL. Signal transducer and activator of transcription-3 (STAT3) is constitutively activated in normal, self-renewing B-1 cells but only inducibly expressed in conventional B lymphocytes. *J Exp Med.* 1997; 185:1035–1042

45. Karras JG, Wang Z, Huo L, Frank DA, Rothstein TL. Induction of STAT protein signaling through the CD40 receptor in B lymphocytes: distinct STAT activation following surface Ig and CD40 receptor engagement. *J Immunol.* 1997;159:4350–4355

46. Majolini MB, D'Elios MM, Galieni P, Boncristiano M, Lauria F, Del Prete G, Telford JL, Baldari CT. Expression of the T-cell-specific tyrosine kinase Lck in normal B-1 cells and in chronic lymphocytic leukemia B cells. *Blood.* 1998;91:3390–3396

47. Kipps TJ, Carson DA. Autoantibodies in chronic lymphocytic leukemia and related systemic autoimmune diseases. *Blood.* 1993;81:2475–2487

48. Fais F, Ghiotto F, Hashimoto S, Sellars B, Valetto A, Allen SL, Schulman P, Vinciguerra VP, Rai K, Rassenti LZ, Kipps TJ, Dighiero G, Schroeder HW, Ferrarini M, Chiorazzi N. Chronic lymphocytic leukemia B cells express restricted sets of mutated and unmutated antigen receptors. *J Clin Invest.* 1998;102:1515–1525

49. Lewis CM, Pegrum GD. Autoimmune antibodies in chronic lymphatic leukaemia. *Br J Haematol.* 1978;38:75–84

50. Hamblin TJ, Oscier DG, Young BJ. Autoimmunity in chronic lymphocytic leukaemia. *J Clin Pathol.* 1986;39:713–716

51. Keller RH, Libnoch, J.A. Kallas G *et al.* Sequential T-cell immunoregulatory subsets and function in B-CLL. In: Gale RP, Rai, K., eds. *Chronic Lymphocytic Leukemia: Recent Progress and Future Directions.* New York: Liss; 1987:147

52. Gonzalez H, Leblond V, Azar N, Sutton L, Gabarre J, Binet JL, Vernant JP, Dighiero G. Severe autoimmune hemolytic anemia in eight patients treated with fludarabine. *Hematol Cell Ther.* 1998;40:113–118

53. Dighiero G. Adverse and beneficial immunological effects of purine nucleoside analogues. *Hematol Cell Ther.* 1996;38 Suppl 2:S75–S81

54. Serrano D, Monteiro J, Allen SL, Kolitz J, Schulman P, Lichtman SM, Buchbinder A, Vinciguerra VP, Chiorazzi N, Gregersen PK. Clonal expansion within the CD4+CD57+ and CD8+CD57+ T cell subsets in chronic lymphocytic leukemia. *J Immunol.* 1997; 158:1482–1489

55. Serrano J, Monteiro J, Allen SI, Kolitz J, Schulman P, Lichtman SM, Buchbinder A, Vinciguerra VP, Chiorazzi N, Gregersen PK. Clonal expansion within the CD+CD57+ T cell subsets in chronic lymphocytic leukemia. *J Immunol.* 1997;158:1482–1489

56. Rutella S, Rumi C, Puggioni P, Barberi T, Di Mario A, Larocca LM, Leone G. Expression of thrombospondin receptor (CD36) in B-cell chronic lymphocytic leukemia as an indicator of tumor cell dissemination. *Haematologica.* 1999;84:419–424

57. Bauvois B, De Meester I, Dumont J, Rouillard D, Zhao HX, Bosmans E. Constitutive expression of CD26/dipeptidylpeptidase IV on peripheral blood B lymphocytes of patients with B chronic lymphocytic leukaemia. *Br J Cancer.* 1999;79:1042–1048

58. Zupo S, Isnardi L, Megna M, Massara R, Malavasi F, Dono M, Cosulich E, Ferrarini M. CD38 expression distinguishes two groups of B-cell chronic lymphocytic leukemias with different responses to anti-IgM antibodies and propensity to apoptosis. *Blood.* 1996;88:1365–1374

59. Eistere W, Hilbe W, Stauder R, Bechter O, Fend F, Thaler J. An aggressive subtype of B-CLL is characterized by strong CD44 expression and lack of CD11c. *Br J Haematol.* 1996;93:661–669

60. Nakamura N, Kuze T, Hashimoto Y, Tasaki K, Hojo H, Sasaki Y, Sato M, Abe M. Analysis of the immunoglobulin heavy chain gene variable region of 101 cases with peripheral B cell neoplasms and B cell chronic lymphocytic leukemia in the Japanese population. *Pathol Int.* 1999;49:595–600

61. Lankester AC, van Schijndel GM, van der Schoot CE, van Oers MH, van Noesel CJ, van Lier RA. Antigen receptor nonresponsiveness in chronic lymphocytic leukemia B cells. *Blood.* 1995;86:1090–1071

62. Alfarano A, Circosta P, Vallario A, Camaschella C, Indraccolo S, Amadori A, Caligaris-Cappio F. Alternative splicing of CD79a (Ig alpha) and CD79b (Ig beta) transcripts in human B-CLL cells. *Curr Top Microbiol Immunol.* 1999;246:241–248

63. Alfarano A, Indraccolo S, Circosta P, Minuzzo S, Vallario A, Zamarchi R, Fregonese A, Calderazzo F, Faldella A, Aragno M, Camaschella C, Amadori A, Caligaris-Cappio F. An alternatively spliced form of CD79b gene may account for altered B-cell receptor expression in B-chronic lymphocytic leukemia. *Blood.* 1999;93:2327–2335

64. Thompson AA, Talley JA, Do HN, Kagan HL, Kunkel L, Berenson J, Cooper MD, Saxon A, Wall R. Aberrations of the B-cell receptor B29 (CD79b) gene in chronic lymphocytic leukemia. *Blood.* 1997;90:1387–1394

65. Burrows PD, Cooper MD. B-cell development and differentiation. *Curr Opin Immunol.* 1997;9:239–244

66. Reed JC. Bcl-2: prevention of apoptosis as a mechanism of drug resistance. *Hematol Oncol Clin North Am.* 1995;9:451–473

67. Reed JC. Regulation of apoptosis by bcl-2 family proteins and its role in cancer and chemoresistance. *Curr Opin Oncol.* 1995;7:541–546

68. Pepper C, Thomas A, Hoy T, Bentley P. Chlorambucil resistance in B-cell chronic lymphocytic leukaemia is mediated through failed Bax induction and selection of high Bcl-2-expressing subclones. *Br J Haematol.* 1999;104:581–588

69. Molica S, Mannella A, Crispino G, Dattilo A, Levato D. Comparative flow cytometric evaluation of bcl-2 oncoprotein in CD5+ and CD5- B-cell lymphoid chronic leukemias. *Haematologica.* 1997;82:555–559

70. Kitada S, Andersen J, Akar S, Zapata JM, Takayama S, Krajewski S, Wang HG, Zhang X, Bullrich F, Croce CM, Rai K, Hines J, Reed JC. Expression of apoptosis-regulating proteins in chronic lymphocytic leukemia: correlations with *in vitro* and *in vivo* chemoresponses. *Blood.* 1998;91:3379–3389

71. Webb A, Cunningham D, Cotter F, Clarke PA, di Stefano F, Ross P, Corbo M, Dziewanowska Z. BCL-2 antisense therapy in patients with non-Hodgkin lymphoma. *Lancet.* 1997; 349:1137–1141

72. Nowell PC, Moore JS. Aberrant responses of human lymphocytic neoplasms to cytokine regulation. *Immunol Res.* 1998;17:171–177

73. Castejon R, Vargas JA, Romero Y, Briz M, Munoz RM, Durantez A. Modulation of apoptosis by cytokines in B-cell chronic lymphocytic leukemia. *Cytometry.* 1999;38:224–230

74. Pu QQ, Bezwoda WR. Interleukin-4 prevents spontaneous in-vitro apoptosis in chronic lymphatic leukaemia but sensitizes B-CLL cells to melphalan cytotoxicity. *Br J Haematol.* 1997;98:413–417

75. Mainou-Fowler T, Prentice AG. Modulation of apoptosis with cytokines in B-cell chronic lymphocytic leukaemia. *Leuk Lymphoma.* 1996;21:369–377

76. Molica S, Vitelli G, Levato D, Levato L, Dattilo A, Gandolfo GM. Clinico-biological implications of increased serum levels of interleukin-8 in B-cell chronic lymphocytic leukemia. *Haematologica.* 1999;84:208–211

77. Konig A, Menzel T, Lynen S, Wrazel L, Rosen A, Al Katib A, Raveche E, Gabrilove JL. Basic fibroblast growth factor (bFGF) upregulates the expression of bcl-2 in B cell chronic lymphocytic leukemia cell lines resulting in delaying apoptosis. *Leukemia.* 1997;11:258–265

78. Nilsson J, Soderberg O, Nilsson K, Rosen A. Thioredoxin prolongs survival of B-type chronic lymphocytic leukemia cells. *Blood.* 2000;95:1420–1426

79. Osorio LM, De Santiago A, Aguilar-Santelises M, Mellstedt H, Jondal M. CD6 ligation modulates the Bcl-2/Bax ratio and protects chronic lymphocytic leukemia B cells from apoptosis induced by anti-IgM. *Blood.* 1997;89:2833–2841

80. Romano MF, Lamberti A, Tassone P, Alfinito F, Costantini S, Chiurazzi F, Defrance T, Bonelli P, Tuccillo F, Turco MC, Venuta S. Triggering of CD40 antigen inhibits fludarabine-induced apoptosis in B chronic lymphocytic leukemia cells [published erratum appears in *Blood* 1999 Mar 15;93(6):2141]. *Blood.* 1998;92:990–995

81. Tangye SG, Raison RL. Human cytokines suppress apoptosis of leukaemic CD5+ B cells and preserve expression of bcl-2. *Immunol Cell Biol.* 1997;75:127–135

82. Rojas R, Roman J, Torres A, Ramirez R, Carracedo J, Lopez R, Garcia JM, Martin C, Pintado O. Inhibition of apoptotic cell death in B-CLL by interferon gamma correlates with clinical stage. *Leukemia.* 1996;10:1782–1788

83. Osorio LM, Aguilar-Santelises M. Apoptosis in B-chronic lymphocytic leukaemia. *Med Oncol.* 1998;15:234–240

84. Chandra J, Gilbreath J, Freireich EJ, Kliche KO, Andreeff M, Keating M, McConkey DJ. Protease activation is required for glucocorticoid-induced apoptosis in chronic lymphocytic leukemic lymphocytes. *Blood.* 1997;90:3673–3681

85. Tangye SG, Weston KM, Raison RL. Interleukin-10 inhibits the *in vitro* proliferation of human activated leukemic CD5+ B-cells. *Leuk Lymphoma.* 1998;31:121–130

86. Sjoberg J, Aguilar-Santelises M, Sjogren AM, Pisa EK, Ljungdahl A, Bjorkholm M, Jondal M, Mellstedt H, Pisa P. Interleukin-10 mRNA expression in B-cell chronic lymphocytic leukaemia inversely correlates with progression of disease. *Br J Haematol.* 1996;92:393–400

87. Trentin L, Zambello R, Facco M, Sancetta R, Agostini C, Semenzato G. Interleukin-15: a novel cytokine with regulatory properties on normal and neoplastic B lymphocytes. *Leuk Lymphoma.* 1997;27:35–42

88. Lagneaux L, Delforge A, Bron D, De Bruyn C, Stryckmans P. Chronic lymphocytic leukemic B cells but not normal B cells are rescued from apoptosis by contact with normal bone marrow stromal cells. *Blood.* 1998;91:2387–2396

89. Martin DA, Zheng L, Siegel RM, Huang B, Fisher GH, Wang J, Jackson CE, Puck JM, Dale J, Straus SE, Peter ME, Krammer PH, Fesik S, Lenardo MJ. Defective CD95/APO-1/Fas signal complex formation in the human autoimmune lymphoproliferative syndrome, type Ia. *Proc Natl Acad Sci USA.* 1999;96:4552–4557

90. Panayiotidis P, Ganeshaguru K, Foroni L, Hoffbrand AV. Expression and function of the FAS antigen in B chronic lymphocytic leukemia and hairy cell leukemia. *Leukemia.* 1995; 9:1227–1232

91. Hennino A, Berard M, Casamayor-Palleja M, Krammer PH, Defrance T. Regulation of the Fas death pathway by FLICE-inhibitory protein in primary human B cells. *J Immunol.* 2000;165:3023–3030

92. Kitada S, Zapata JM, Andreeff M, Reed JC. Bryostatin and CD40-ligand enhance apoptosis resistance and induce expression of cell survival genes in B-cell chronic lymphocytic leukaemia. *Br J Haematol.* 1999;106:995–1004

93. Tinhofer I, Marschitz I, Kos M, Henn T, Egle A, Villunger A., Greil R. Differential sensitivity of CD4+ and CD8+ T lymphocytes to the killing efficacy of Fas (Apo-1/CD95) ligand+ tumor cells in B chronic lymphocytic leukemia. *Blood.* 1998;91:4273-81

94. Osorio LM, Jondal M, Aguilar-Santelises M. Regulation of B-CLL apoptosis through membrane receptors and Bcl-2 family proteins. *Leuk Lymphoma.* 1998;30:247–256

95. De Rossi G, Marroni P, Paganuzzi M, Mauro FR, Tenca C, Zarcone D, Velardi A, Molica S, Grossi CE. Increased serum levels of soluble CD44 standard, but not of variant isoforms v5 and v6, in B cell chronic lymphocytic leukemia. *Leukemia.* 1997;11:134–141

96. Illges H, Braun M, Peter HH, Melchers I. Analysis of the human CD21 transcription unit reveals differential splicing of exon 11 in mature transcripts and excludes alternative splicing as the mechanism causing solubilization of CD21. *Mol Immunol.* 1997;34:683–693

97. Molica S, Vitelli G, Levato D, Crispino G, Dell'Olio M, Dattilo A, Matera R, Gandolfo GM, Musto P. CD27 in B-cell chronic lymphocytic leukemia. Cellular expression, serum release and correlation with other soluble molecules belonging to nerve growth factor receptors (NGFr) superfamily. *Haematologica.* 1998;83:398–408

98. Callea V, Morabito F, Oliva BM, Stelitano C, Levato D, Dattilo A, Gangemi F, Iorfida A, Iacopino P, Nobile F, Molica S, Brugiatelli M. Surface CD14 positivity in B-cell chronic lymphocytic leukaemia is related to clinical outcome. *Br J Haematol.* 1999;107:347–352

99. Molica S, Levato D, Dell'Olio M, Matera R, Minervini M, Dattilo A, Carotenuto M, Musto P. Cellular expression and serum circulating levels of CD23 in B-cell chronic lymphocytic leukemia. Implications for prognosis. *Haematologica.* 1996;81:428–433

100. Knauf WU, Langenmayer I, Ehlers B, Mohr B, Adorf D, Nerl CH, Hallek M, Zwingers TH, Emmerich B, Thiel E. Serum levels of soluble CD23, but not soluble CD25, predict disease progression in early stage B-cell chronic lymphocytic leukemia. *Leuk Lymphoma.* 1997; 27:523–532

101. Desablens B, Garidi R, Tabuteau S, Capiod JC, Fuentes V, Lassoued K. Biological or clinical parameters for assessment of prognosis in B-CCL? Analysis of 156 patients *Blood* 2000; 96: (abstract 4916)

102. EORTC Leukemia Cooperative Group. A randomized Phase II trial of high-dose chlorambucil vs. fludarabine in patients with advanced B-chronic lymphocytic leukemia. *Hematol Cell Ther.* 1999;41:127–136

2

The Road to Remission: From Single Agent Intervention to Combination Therapy and Onward

Leukemia and lymphoma treatment has been at the forefront of tumor chemotherapy development for the last quarter of a century, because compared with treatment of solid tumors, delivery to the site of action presents fewer difficulties. However, the unique nature of B-CLL presents its own problems, with its accumulation of slowly proliferating but long-lived lymphocytes. Purging methods which rely on intervention with the metabolism of the cell, in growth or in the stimulation of programmed cell death, are likely to leave behind a small number of refractory cells, resting in G_0 and so impervious to outside factors. These cells will eventually repopulate the blood and marrow, causing relapse. Treated cells also develop methods of drug resistance, so that patients become refractory to re-treatment with multiple courses of the same drug.

In the past decade a large number of regimens have been trialled without substantially altering outcome. While a substantial number of patients respond to chemotherapy, relapse is almost inevitable.

As new agents for therapy are developed and fully assessed, the trend is for a single agent to be established as efficacious, then used as the basis of combination therapies, until a more powerful single agent emerges with unequivocal advantages. Then it, in its turn, is used as a basis for novel combination therapies. A general algorithm for treatment of B-CLL is shown in Figure 1.

In general, new therapies prove themselves capable of producing remissions when used as second- or third-line treatment. They are then incorporated into treatment of disease earlier in its course.

The effort to increase remissions began with traditional management using the alkylating agent chlorambucil, and on occasion combined it

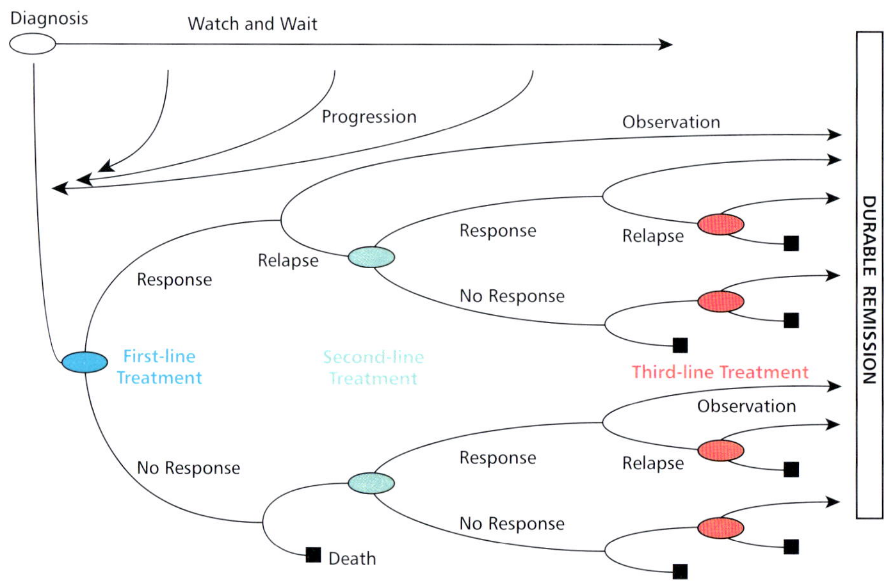

Figure 1. General CLL treatment algorithm

with steroids, cross-linking agents, and purine analogues. Treatment has shifted so that the purine analogue fludarabine is the single agent of choice, to be used in combination with other chemotherapies, monoclonal antibodies and other novel therapies.

Chlorambucil: alkylating agent of choice in B-CLL: mode of action

- Forms covalent bonds with N-7 of guanine in DNA
- Nitrogen mustard family of alkylating agents
- Not cell-cycle-phase-specific
- Tumor resistance probably due to enhanced DNA repair
- Mutagenic: long-term therapy may induce secondary malignancies
- May produce cumulative myelosuppression

A substantial body of data acquired using chlorambucil (CLB) to treat CLL has established that there is no survival advantage in using this alkylating agent on patients with early disease (Binet stage A, Rai stage I)[1] and that an intermittent regimen has less hematological toxicity than a continuous regimen[2]. The addition of the glucocorticoid methyl-prednisolone (prednisone)[3] further ameliorates myelosuppression which is of particular importance when the patient has presented with pure red cell aplasia, auto-immune hemolytic anemia or thrombocytopenia. A short course of prednisone may be used as frontline therapy in such patients with low red cell and platelet counts. In addition to their myelosuppressive effects, alkylating agents, when used in continuous regimens such as in the CLL-80 trial, may also induce secondary malignancies[4].

In general, the overall response rate with CLB-based regimens has been between 40% and 60%, with complete responses in less that 20% of patients[5]. The most common and least myelosuppressive regimen is intermittent dosage of 20–40 mg/m^2 every 2 weeks, but produces only moderate responses. High-dose continuous administration of CLB[6] is more effective and is under investigation in trials of flexible design which allow moderation of dosage in response to toxicity[7]. The alternative alkylating agent, cyclophosphamide, inactive until it has been metabolized by cytochrome P450 in the liver, provides an alternative for patients unable to tolerate CLB, and, because it is absorbed as an inert compound, is used extensively in combination therapies. Cyclophosphamide can be given both orally and intravenously, under a wide range of dosing regimens, according to patient response and other therapy. While it is generally given as a large i.v. dose divided over several days, it may also be scheduled with relatively small doses given more frequently on a continuous basis. High-dose cyclophosphamide (up to 120 mg/kg) is also used as part of combination therapy as a conditioning regimen that precedes bone marrow transplantation.

Cyclophosphamide: mode of action

- Activated by cytochrome P450 microsomal oxidase system
- Converted to aldophosphamide (nitrogen mustard) and acrolein (no anti-tumor effects)
- Not cell-cycle-phase-specific
- Tumor resistance probably due to enhanced DNA repair.
- Mutagenic: long-term therapy may induce secondary malignancies

- Additional toxicities due to acrolein: bladder toxicity, hemorrhagic cystitis)
- Adequate hydration essential

A number of multi-drug combinations have been assessed using compounds whose action could be additive or synergistic with these alkylating agents.

These regimens include:

- CMP (cyclophosphamide, melphalan, prednisone)[8]
- CAP (cyclophosphamide, doxorubicin, prednisone)[9]
- COP (cyclophosphamide, vincristine, prednisone[10]
- CHOP (cyclophosphamide, hydroxyldaunomycin, vincristine, prednisone)[6,11,12]

None of these trials has shown convincing improvements when compared to chlorambucil with or without prednisone, and some of the anthracyclines such as doxorubicin (adriamycin) are no longer considered effective in B-CLL.

Doxorubicin (adriamycin) and **daunomycin: mode of action**

- Anthracycline antibiotics: glycoside bound to an amino sugar
- Intercalate into DNA
- Inhibit topoisomerase II

Vincristine (oncovin): **mode of action**

- Microtubule assembly inhibitor
- Derived from rosy periwinkle *Vinca rosea*
- S-phase-specific

Many other single agents, such as IFN-α[13,14] chlorambucil[15] and IL-2[16] have been assessed in B-CLL with moderate or no clinical effect.

Purine analogues

The group of agents which most fulfill their promise in B-CLL are the purine analogues, particularly the soluble fluorinated compound, fludarabine phosphate. The three most intensively investigated purine analogue structures, are shown in Figure 2.

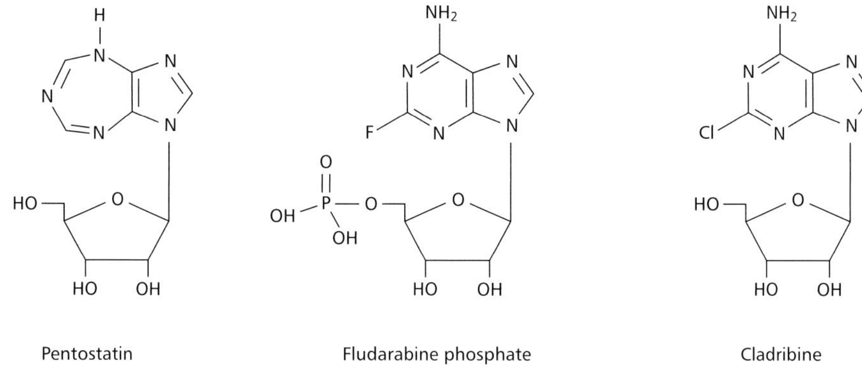

Figure 2. Structure of purine analogues

While the structures of these nucleoside analogues are very similar, they do not all act in precisely the same way and have been found to show different clinical efficacies. Pentostatin (deoxycoformycin, DCF) is primarily an inhibitor of adenosine deaminase. Cladribine (2-CdA) and fludarabine (F-AMP) have multiple inhibitory activities within the cell, not all of which have been fully characterized. Figure 3 shows purine analogue metabolic pathways and some of the pathways they inhibit.

Pentostatin

Further processing of deoxycoformycin (pentostatin) within the cell is not required for activity. It acts directly as a potent inhibitor of adenosine deaminase, an enzyme required for deoxyadenosine breakdown and elimination. This causes dATP to accumulate to toxic levels and is active in non-replicating lymphoid cells[17]. It has proved to be an effective agent in hairy cell leukemia (HCL) but appears less effective against B-CLL, with overall response and complete response in pre-treated patients lower than after treatment with fludarabine[18]. As yet, it has rarely been used as an agent of first-line defence in B-CLL.

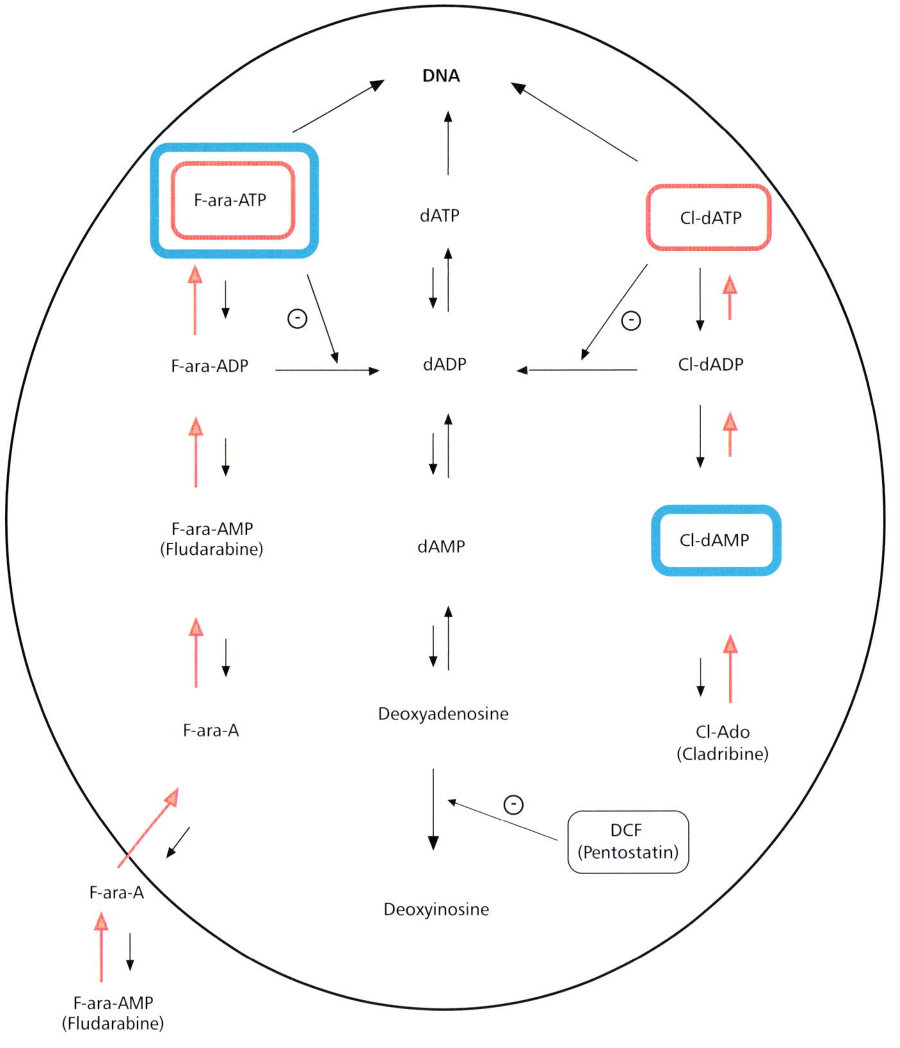

Figure 3. Metabolism and action of purine analogues

Cladribine

The metabolite of cladribine which accumulates to highest levels within the cell is the monophosphate shown in blue in Figure 3. The active metabolite, however, is the triphosphate, shown in red, and since this has a rapid turnover, frequent administration of cladribine is necessary for optimal effectiveness. Cladribine has, therefore, been extensively evaluated for routes of administration other than by intravenous infusion, and while oral availability is only a third of infusion levels[19], subcutaneous injections produce a plasma levels equivalent to infusion[20].

DNA synthesis in growing cells is inhibited after administration by two distinct mechanisms. Cl-dATP inhibits DNA polymerases, becoming incorporated into the DNA but more slowly than dATP, causing pausing and stuttering of the polymerase complex. Cladribine is also a potent inhibitor of ribonucleotide reductase, further disrupting nucleotide balances, and therefore DNA synthesis and repair, within the replicating cell[21].

Fludarabine

Fludarabine phosphate is rapidly dephosphorylated by serum enzymes, transported into the cell as the nucleoside and rephosphorylated within the cell, with none of these steps being rate limiting. It then has the advantage that the metabolite which accumulates within the cell, rapidly achieving active levels after administration, is the active metabolite, F-ara-ATP[22]. This nucleoside triphosphate has multiple activities within the cell, some of which are shared to some extent by cladribine, some of which are unique (Table1).

Table 1. Actions of F-ara-ATP

Actions of F ara-ATP	Effect on:
• Competes with dATP for incorporation into DNA	• DNA polymerases • DNA primase
• Resistant to removal	• DNA polymerase exonuclease activity
• Chain terminator	• DNA polymerase • DNA ligase
• Promotes double-strand breaks	• Apoptosis
• Inhibits RNA synthesis	• RNA polymerase
• Substrate-limiting for DNA repair	• Ribonucleotide reductase

It inhibits DNA synthesis by competing with normal nucleotides for incorporation into replicating strands by the polymerase complex.

Once incorporated, F-ara-A is an effective chain terminator, producing single- and double-strand breaks, inhibiting DNA ligase, producing DNA deletions and mutations, and promoting apoptosis. It also effectively inhibits ribonucleotide reductase, disrupting DNA repair by reducing the amounts of available deoxynucleotides. Fludarabine-induced apoptosis is not restricted to proliferating cells and is the main method of lymphocytic cell death.

Uniquely, F-ara-C can inhibit RNA synthesis, which may be the mechanism behind its action on resting as well as proliferating lymphocytes. This inhibition, which appears to act by incorporation of fludarabine into mRNA terminating transcription, has been recently shown to correlate significantly with the cytotoxicity of fludarabine in B-CLL[23]. It is suggested that cell death occurs due to a preferential depletion of short-lived proteins. The combination of fludarabine with compounds capable of inhibiting protein synthesis directly, such as cycloheximide, may prove a useful therapeutic approach in the treatment of B-CLL[24].

Purine analogue-related toxicity

The main complications of treatment with purine analogues lie in their myelosuppressive and immunosuppressive potential. The most common side-effect is granulocytopenia, but this is not cumulative and usually subsides in the course of treatment. T-cell suppression is cumulative, and is particularly pronounced with pentostatin and cladribine, since CD4 cells remain decreased for several years following cessation of treatment[25]. Opportunistic infections (by organisms including *Candida,* herpes, *Listeria* and *Legionella*) due to long-lasting T-cell suppression have proved a problem with cladribine[26-28], some of the regimens of fludarabine[29] and pentostatin[25]. Opportunistic infections occur less often when purine analogues are given as frontline agents. These agents are typically administered as outpatient therapy. However, when the patient has a large tumor mass and responds rapidly, the first cycle of treatment may cause acute renal toxicity due to tumor lysis syndrome, so initial treatment must take place where the patient can be monitored.

These analogues are also potentially mutagenic, both directly due to their incorporation into DNA and indirectly due to their myelosuppressive effects, which may facilitate tumor evasion of immune surveillance. An investigation to establish the rates of such secondary malignancies reviewed the data for 2014 patients treated on National Cancer Institute Group C protocols[30]. Fludarabine was used for relapsed and refractory CLL (n=724). DCF and/or CdA was used for hairy cell leukemia (HCL, total patients, n=1290, DCF, n=409, CdA, n=979). The numbers of observed and expected secondary tumors were compared. They observed 111 malignancies ranging from lymphoma (25 patients), prostate (19), lung (15), colorectal (nine), bladder (six) and breast (six patients) cancers, with individual cases of cancer affecting the CNS, stomach, ovary, head and neck, melanoma, sarcoma, testes and myeloid cells. Comparison with age-adjusted 1994 Surveillance and Epidemiology End-Results rates for the general population, the observed/expected frequencies for DCF, fludarabine, and CdA were 1.43 (95% confidence interval [CI], 0.93–2.10), 1.65 (95% CI, 1.04–2.47), and 1.50 (95% CI, 1.14–1.93), respectively, indicating a significant ($p = 0.05$) increase in risk for patients treated on the latter two protocols compared with a normal population. However, these values were found to be consistent with the increase already associated with these diseases, and the authors concluded that these analogues do not significantly increase the risk of secondary malignancies.

Purine analogues in trials

Most of the trials involving pentostatin have been on previously treated patients[17,18] and while it has produced good responses in HCL, it seems to be less active in CLL than fludarabine[31], producing fewer complete responses and shorter remissions.

Fludarabine has now been extensively assessed in a large number of trials in the last decade, while cladribine results are fewer and less mature. In general, cladribine remissions are impressive but short-lived[32]. Treatment results of major trials using fludarabine and cladribine are shown in Table 2 (updated and expanded from Kalil and Cheson, 1999)[33].

Fludarabine as single agent compares very favorably with trials using intermittent dosage of chlorambucil and is currently under investigation to compare short intravenous courses of fludarabine with high-dose chlorambucil[7]. Its efficacy as an orally administered agent is also under investigation[34].

Table 2. Fludarabine and cladribine activity in B-CLL

Fludarabine					Cladribine				
Ref	**Patients (*n*)**	**OR (%)**	**CR (%)**	**Duration (months)**	**Ref**	**Patients (*n*)**	**OR (%)**	**CR (%)**	**Duration (months)**
Salvage agent					**Salvage agent**				
35	32	13	3	NA	36	90	44	4	4
37	169	52	37	22					
38	78	58	14	21	39	26	31	0	1640
40	42	31	0	6	41	92	36	5	NA
42	18	67	NA	6	43	52	58	31	20
44	20	55	20	NA	45	19	68	11	9+**
46	13	62	15	28	41	184	12.5	48.5	13.5
47	21	48	5	NA					
9	48								
48		48	13	11					
Frontline agent					**Frontline agent**				
38	35	80	37	33	49	20	85	10	8+**
37	95	71	23	24+**	32	19	74	47	NA*
9	52	70	27	34+**	19	63	75	16	14
50	170	63	20	25	51	30	80	20	NA*
46	25	92	40	33+**	41	194	82.5	45.5	14.7
52	16	100	31	NA					

NA, information not available
CR, complete response
OR, overall responses (PR+CR)
+** median duration not yet reached

Fludarabine first established itself as a salvage agent capable of inducing responses in otherwise refractory disease[29,48,53,54]. Several major randomized trials have now compared the efficacy of fludarabine to alkylating agent-based chemotherapy as frontline treatment. One major trial was the CALGB, Southwest Oncology Group (SWOG), Cancer Therapy Group/National Cancer Institute of Canada (CTG/NCI), and Eastern Cooperative Oncology Group (ECOG) intergroup study[50]. In this study 509 untreated patients with active disease were allocated to receive fludarabine (25 mg/m^2/day for 5 days) or CLB (40 mg/m^2/day 1) or a combination of fludarabine and CLB (20 mg/m^2 of each drug, CLB on day 1, fludarabine days 1–5) every 4 weeks for up to 12 months. Patients who failed to respond or who experienced progressive disease with the original treatment in the first 6 months, were crossed over to the other arm. The 170 patients from the fludarabine group had an overall response rate of 63% (20% complete response (CR) and 43% partial response (PR)). This was significantly higher ($p < 0.001$) than the overall response rate of 37% (4% CR and 33% PR) seen in the 181 patients from the CLB group. The duration of response was also significantly longer in the fludarabine group, 25 months versus 14 months for those in the CLB group ($p = 0.001$). Survival analysis for 507 patients was available. The median progression-free survival was 20 months for the fludarabine group and 14 months for the CLB group ($p < 0.001$). However, no difference in overall survival (66 months with fludarabine versus 56 months with CLB) was seen at a median follow-up of 62 months.

The French Cooperative Group on CLL[9,55] evaluated 695 previously untreated stage B (486) and C (209) patients; 225 received fludarabine (25 mg/m^2/day), or one of two anthracycline-based standard combination regimens: 238 patients received CAP, and 232 patients received CHOP. Histological remission (HR) and immunological remission (IR) were defined as normal BM biopsy and <100 CD5+/CD19+ cells/μl in the peripheral blood. HR was 24%, 8%, 24%, respectively; partial remission, defined as greater than 50% reduction of measurable disease manifestations and a more than 50% improvement of all abnormal blood counts, was 49%, 53%, 44%, respectively; and failure was 23%, 35%, and 19%, respectively, for the CHOP, CAP, and fludarabine groups. Clinical and hematological remission (CHR) was observed in 37% of fludarabine, 28% of CHOP, and 13% in the CAP group. In the fludarabine, CHOP, and CAP groups, IR was 55%, 35% and 29%, respectively, and the numbers of reported deaths were 38, 51, and 62, respectively.

In previously treated patients, fludarabine is most effectively used in 5-day schedules, 25 to 30 mg/m^2/day[44]. Other schedules have explored once-a-week fludarabine and a 3-day schedule every 4 weeks. These strategies, in particular the once-a-week schedule, have obtained inferior results[40]. The addition of prednisone has not been associated with an improvement in response rate or survival.

Some of the smaller scale trials of both untreated and previously treated B-CLL where retrospective analysis was undertaken to clarify the role of the drug, have produced impressive responses to fludarabine[56]. In this recent analysis, 47 patients affected by advanced CLL; 36% untreated, 31.9% relapsed and 31.9% resistant, had been treated with fludarabine at 25 mg/m^2/day, either for 4 days every 3 weeks in 29 cases, or for 5 days every 4 weeks in 18. The median number of fludarabine cycles was six (range 2–11). Response was defined according to total tumor mass (TTM), score reduction and toxicity was expressed according to WHO grading criteria and the median follow-up of the series was 13 months from the beginning of therapy. The response rate was 74.4%, with 34% complete response (CR). The overall response rate was 94%, 80% and 46.6% in untreated, relapsed and resistant cases, respectively, and a significantly higher number of responses was associated with no previous treatment and number of fludarabine cycles. Fifty-three per cent of all cases and 58.8% of untreated ones did not experience any toxicity. Treatment-related side-effects were mainly autoimmune phenomena in untreated patients and infectious complications in treated ones. One heavily pre-treated patient died because of neurologic complications. Median time to re-treatment was 18 months (range 1–30) and was influenced by age and previous treatment. The overall median survival was 35.7 months with a significantly higher proportion of surviving cases among Rai 0–II stages, responders and patients receiving more than five fludarabine cycles.

While not all patient cohorts respond so comprehensively or with so few adverse events to fludarabine treatment, fludarabine achieves more responses than any other single agent currently in use.

To date, no treatment combination has given better results in large-scale trials than fludarabine alone.

Nevertheless, no chemotherapy regimen has yet clearly prolonged survival in CLL, and so smaller Phase II trials are underway adding other agents to fludarabine, with promising results in responses and duration of remission.

Based on an *in vitro* synergy between fludarabine and anthracyclines, a regimen of combined fludarabine and epirubicin has been used in a German multicenter Phase II study of 38 patients with advanced CLL[46], 25 of whom were previously untreated. The overall response (OR) was 82%, with 32% achieving complete responses. The previously untreated group showed OR of 95% and CR of 42%, while patients who had previously received alkylating agents showed an OR of 62% and a CR of 15%. Responses were also early in treatment; 12 patients responding immediately to the first cycle, another six after the second and another 11 after the third. Median remission duration was 19 months (7–37 months), with 15 patients still in ongoing remission.

The anthracenedione mitoxantrone, which was discovered in the search for less toxic doxorubicin analogues, has been successfully used in non-Hodgkin's lymphoma. Marked immunosuppression limited mitoxantrone's efficacy when used in combination with fludarabine and dexamethasone[57]. When mitoxantrone is combined with fludarabine without dexamethasone[58], the regimen is tolerated reasonably well and is effective. The results on 25 patients, 12 of whom had been previously untreated, showed 100% response in the untreated cohort, including 40% CR. However, this combination does not appear to give a survival advantage.

A phase I study which used fludarabine in combination with cyclophosphamide[7], on untreated patients also obtained 100% response, with 89% a complete response. Median overall and disease-free survival times had not been reached at the 5-year time point.

Such studies have confirmed the efficacy of fludarabine as a frontline agent and continue to show improvements in numbers and duration of clinical responses.

Assessment of response at the molecular level may show residual clonal malignant cells remain, even when there is no longer evidence of clinical disease[51]. Molecular remissions form a subset of clinical remissions obtained with fludarabine[58] and are associated with a better outcome, particularly when the patients in remission are treated by bone marrow transplantation.

However, the problem remains in B-CLL that most patients do eventually relapse, and while fludarabine-containing regimens have been shown to be partially successful as salvage therapy even when fludarabine was used as frontline therapy, some patients became refractory. In addition, patients who have received other chemotherapy regimens may never respond to fludarabine at all.

There are two interrelated approaches showing particular promise to supplement chemotherapy in B-CLL. Achievement of even short-term responses can allow treatment by bone marrow transplantation. In addition, another approach to remission may be using monoclonal antibody therapy which depletes the blood and marrow of cells bearing significant markers. Campath-1H, a humanized antibody which recognises the CD52 antigen is an example of a monoclonal which has the ability to supplement or possibly replace existing chemotherapy regimens.

Reference List

1. Shustik C, Mick R, Silver R, Sawitsky A, Rai K, Shapiro L. Treatment of early chronic lymphocytic leukemia: intermittent chlorambucil versus observation. *Hematol Oncol.* 1988;6:7–12

2. Jaksic B, Brugiatelli M. High-dose continuous chlorambucil vs intermittent chlorambucil plus prednisone for treatment of B-CLL: IGCI CLL-01 trial. *Nouv Rev Fr Hematol* 1988;30:437-442

3. Keller JW, Knospe WH, Raney M, Huguley CMJ, Johnson L, Bartolucci AA, Omura GA. Treatment of chronic lymphocytic leukemia using chlorambucil and prednisone with or without cycle-active consolidation chemotherapy. A Southeastern Cancer Study Group Trial. *Cancer.* 1986;58:1185–1192

4. Dighiero G, Maloum K, Desablens B, Cazin B, Navarro M, Leblay R, Leporrier M, Jaubert J, Lepeu G, Dreyfus B, Binet JL, Travade P. Chlorambucil in indolent chronic lymphocytic leukemia. French Cooperative Group on Chronic Lymphocytic Leukemia. *N Engl J Med.* 1998;338:1506–1514

5. Sawitsky A, Rai KR, Glidewell O, Silver RT. Comparison of daily versus intermittent chlorambucil and prednisone therapy in the treatment of patients with chronic lymphocytic leukemia. *Blood.* 1977;50:1049–1059

6. Jaksic B, Brugiatelli M, Krc I, Losonczi H, Holowiecki J, Planinc-Peraica A, Kusec R, Morabito F, Iacopino P, Lutz D. High dose chlorambucil versus Binet's modified cyclophosphamide, doxorubicin, vincristine, and prednisone regimen in the treatment of patients with advanced B-cell chronic lymphocytic leukemia. Results of an international multicenter randomized trial. International Society for Chemo-Immunotherapy, Vienna. *Cancer.* 1997;79:2107–2114

7. EORTC Leukemia Cooperative Group. A randomized phase II trial of high-dose chlorambucil vs fludarabine in patients with advanced B-chronic lymphocytic leukemia. *Hematol Cell Ther.* 1999;41:127–136

8. Montserrat E, Alcala A, Alonso C, Besalduch J, Moraleda JM, Garcia-Conde J, Gutierrez M, Gomis F, Garijo J, Guzman MC, *et al.* A randomized trial comparing chlorambucil plus prednisone vs cyclophosphamide, melphalan, and prednisone in the treatment of chronic lymphocytic leukemia stages B and C. *Nouv Rev Fr Hematol.* 1988;30:429–432

9. Johnson S, Smith AG, Loffler H, Osby E, Juliusson G, Emmerich B, Wyld PJ, Hiddemann W. Multicentre prospective randomised trial of fludarabine versus cyclophosphamide, doxorubicin, and prednisone (CAP) for treatment of advanced-stage chronic lymphocytic leukaemia. The French Cooperative Group on CLL. *Lancet.* 1996;347:1432–1438.

10. Montserrat E, Alcala A, Parody R, Domingo A, Garcia-Conde J, Bueno J, Ferran C, Sanz MA, Giralt M, Rubio D, *et al.* Treatment of chronic lymphocytic leukemia in advanced stages. A randomized trial comparing chlorambucil plus prednisone versus cyclophosphamide, vincristine, and prednisone. *Cancer.* 1985;56:2369–2375

11. Binet JL. Treatment of chronic lymphocytic leukaemia. French Co-operative Group on CLL. *Baillieres Clin Haematol.* 1993;6:867–878

12. Is the CHOP regimen a good treatment for advanced CLL? Results from two randomized clinical trials. French Cooperative Group on Chronic Lymphocytic Leukemia. *Leuk Lymphoma.* 1994;13:449–456

13. Misset JL, Mathe G, Gastiaburu J, Goutner A, Dorval T, Gouveia J, Schwarzenberg L, Machover D, Ribaud P, de Vassal F. [Treatment of leukemias and lymphomas by interferons: II. Phase II of the trial treatment of chronic lymphoid leukemia by human interferon alpha+]. *Biomed Pharmacother.* 1982;36:112–116

14. Langenmayer I, Nerl C, Knauf W, Dempster S, Hallek M, Adorf D, Dietzfelbinger H, Busch R, Ziegler-Heitbrock HW, Thiel E, Emmerich B. Interferon-alpha 2b (IFN alpha) for early-phase chronic lymphocytic leukaemia with high risk for disease progression: results of a randomized multicentre study. *Br J Haematol.* 1996;94:362–369

15. Pegourie-Bandelier B, Sotto JJ, Hollard D, Bolla M, Sarrazin R. Therapy program for patients with advanced stages of chronic lymphocytic leukemia. Chlorambucil, splenectomy, and total lymph node irradiation. *Cancer.* 1995;75:2853–2861

16. Allison MA, Jones SE, McGuffey P. Phase II trial of outpatient IL-2 in malignant lymphoma, chronic lymphocytic leukemia, and selected solid tumors. *J Clin Oncol.* 1989;7:75-80

17. Johnson SA, Catovsky D, Child JA, Newland AC, Milligan DW, Janmohamed R. Phase I/II evaluation of pentostatin (2'-deoxycoformycin) in a five day schedule for the treatment of relapsed/refractory B-cell chronic lymphocytic leukaemia. *Invest New Drugs.* 1998;16:155–160

18. Dillman RO, Mick R, McIntyre OR. Pentostatin in chronic lymphocytic leukemia: a phase II trial of Cancer and Leukemia group B. *J Clin Oncol.* 1989;7:433–438

19. Juliusson G, Christiansen I, Hansen MM, Johnson S, Kimby E, Elmhorn-Rosenborg A, Liliemark J. Oral cladribine as primary therapy for patients with B-cell chronic lymphocytic leukemia. *J Clin Oncol.* 1996;14:2160–2166

20. Robak T, Blasinska-Morawiec M, Blonski JZ, Krykowski E, Komarnicki M, Trepinska E, Kazmierczuk M, Hansz J, Dmoszynska A, Rolinski J, Konopka L, Skotnicki AB, Nowak WS, Kotlarek-Haus S, Zdziarska B, Urasinski I. The effect of 2-h infusion of 2-chlorodeoxyadenosine (cladribine) with prednisone in previously untreated B-cell chronic lymphocytic leukaemia. *Eur J Cancer.* 1997;33:2347–2351

21. Plunkett W, Gandhi V. Pharmacology of purine nucleoside analogues. *Hematol Cell Ther.* 1996;38 Suppl 2:S67–S74

22. Gandhi V, Kemena A, Keating MJ, Plunkett W. Cellular pharmacology of fludarabine triphosphate in chronic lymphocytic leukemia cells during fludarabine therapy. *Leuk Lymphoma.* 1993;10:49–56

23. Huang P, Sandoval A, Vand Den Neste E, Keating MJ, Plunkett W. Inhibition of RNA transcription: a biochemical mechanism of action against chronic lymphocytic leukemia cells by fludarabine. *Leukemia.* 2000;14:1405–1413

24. Collins RJ, Harmon BV, Souvlis T, Pope JH, Kerr JF. Effect of cycloheximide on B-chronic lymphocytic leukemia and normal lymphocytes *in vitro*: induction of apoptosis. *Br J Cancer.* 1991;64:518–522

25. Cheson BD. Infectious and immunosuppressive complications of PA therapy. *J Clin Oncol.* 1995;13:2431–2448

26. Betticher DC, Fey MF, von Rohr A, Tobler A, Jenzer H, Gratwohl A, Lohri A, Pugin P, Hess U, Pagani O, *et al.* High incidence of infections after 2-chlorodeoxyadenosine (2-CDA) therapy in patients with malignant lymphomas and chronic and acute leukaemias. *Ann Oncol.* 1994;5:57–64

27. Betticher DC, Ratschiller D, Hsu Schmitz SF, von Rohr A, Hess U, Zulian G, Wernli M, Tichelli A, Tobler A, Fey MF, Cerny T. Reduced dose of subcutaneous cladribine induces identical response rates but decreased toxicity in pretreated chronic lymphocytic leukaemia. Swiss Group for Clinical Cancer Research (SAKK). *Ann Oncol.* 1998;9:721–726

28. Brugiatelli M, Holowiecka B, Dmoszynska A, Krieger O, Planinc-Peraica A, Labar B, Callea V, Morabito F, Jaksic B, Holowiecki J, Lutz D. 2-Chlorodeoxyadenosine treatment in non-Hodgkin's lymphoma and B-cell chronic lymphocytic leukemia resistant to conventional chemotherapy: results of a multicentric experience. International Society for Chemo-Immunotherapy. *Ann Hematol.* 1996;73:79–84

29. Fenchel K, Bergmann L, Wijermans P, Engert A, Pralle H, Mitrou PS, Diehl V, Hoelzer D. Clinical experience with fludarabine and its immunosuppressive effects in pretreated chronic lymphocytic leukemias and low-grade lymphomas. *Leuk Lymphoma.* 1995;18:485–492

30. Cheson BD, Vena DA, Barrett J, Freidlin B. Second malignancies as a consequence of nucleoside analog therapy for chronic lymphoid leukemias. *J Clin Oncol.* 1999;17:2454–2460

31. Grever MR, Leiby JM, Kraut EH, Wilson HE, Neidhart JA, Wall RL, Balcerzak SP. Low-dose deoxycoformycin in lymphoid malignancy. *J Clin Oncol.* 1985;3:1196–1201

32. Delannoy A, Martiat P, Gala JL, Deneys V, Ferrant A, Bosly A, Schieff JM, Michaux JL. 2-Chlorodeoxyadenosine (CdA) for patients with previously untreated chronic lymphocytic leukemia (CLL). *Leukemia.* 1995;9:1130–1135

33. Kalil N, Cheson BD. Chronic lymphocytic leukemia. *The Oncologist.* 1999;4:352–369

34. Foran JM, Oscier D, Orchard J, Johnson SA, Tighe M, Cullen MH, de Takats PG, Kraus C, Klein M, Lister TA. Pharmacokinetic study of single doses of oral fludarabine phosphate in patients with low-grade non-Hodgkin's lymphoma and B-cell chronic lymphocytic leukemia. *J Clin Oncol.* 1999;17:1574–1579

35. Grever MR, Kopecky KJ, Coltman CA, *et al.* Fludarabine monophosphate: a potentially useful agent in chronic lymphocytic leukemia. *Nouv Rev Fr Hematol.* 1998;30:457–459

36. Robak T, Blasinka-Morawiec M, Krykowski E, Kasznicki M, Pluzanska A, Potemski P, Hellmann A, Zaucha JM, Lewandowski K, Dmoszynska A, Hansz J, Komarnicki M, Konopka L, Durzynski T, Ceglarek B, Sikorska A, Kotlarek-Haus S, Mazur G, Urasinski I, Zdziarska B, Maj S, Kopec I, Skotnicki AB, Dwilewicz-Trojaczek J, Grieb P, *et al.* Intermittent 2-hour intravenous infusions of 2-chlorodeoxyadenosine in the treatment of 110 patients with refractory or previously untreated B-cell chronic lymphocytic leukemia. *Leuk Lymphoma.* 1996;22:509–514

37. O'Brien S, Kantarjian H, Beran M, Smith T, Koller C, Estey E, Robertson LE, Lerner S, Keating M. Results of fludarabine and prednisone therapy in 264 patients with chronic lymphocytic leukemia with multivariate analysis-derived prognostic model for response to treatment. *Blood.* 1993;82:1695–1700

38. Keating MJ, O'Brien S, Lerner S, Koller C, Beran M, Robertson LE, Freireich EJ, Estey E, Kantarjian H. Long-term follow-up of patients with chronic lymphocytic leukemia (CLL) receiving fludarabine regimens as initial therapy. *Blood.* 1998;92:1165–1171

39. Tallman MS, Hakimian D, Zanzig C, Hogan DK, Rademaker A, Rose E, Variakojis D. Cladribine in the treatment of relapsed or refractory chronic lymphocytic leukemia. *J Clin Oncol.* 1995;13:983–988

40. Puccio CA, Mittelman A, Lichtman SM, Silver RT, Budman DR, Ahmed T, Feldman EJ, Coleman M, Arnold PM, Arlin ZA, *et al.* A loading dose/continuous infusion schedule of fludarabine phosphate in chronic lymphocytic leukemia. *J Clin Oncol.* 1991;9:1562–1569

41 Robak T, Blonski JZ, Kasznicki M, Konopka L, Ceglarek B, Dmoszynska A, Soroka-Wojtaszko M, Skotnicki AB, Nowak W, Dwilewicz-Trojaczek J, Tomaszewska A, Hellmann A, Lewandowski K, Kuliczkowski K, Potoczek S, Zdziarska B, Hansz J, Kroll R, Komarnicki M, Holowiecki J, Grieb P. Cladribine with or without prednisone in the treatment of previously treated and untreated B-cell chronic lymphocytic leukaemia - updated results of the multicentre study of 378 patients. *Br J Haematol.* 2000;108:357–368

42. Bergmann L, Fenchel K, Jahn B, Mitrou PS, Hoelzer D. Immunosuppressive effects and clinical response of fludarabine in refractory chronic lymphocytic leukemia. *Ann Oncol.* 1993;4:371–375

43. Juliusson G, Liliemark J. Long-term survival following cladribine (2-chlorodeoxyadenosine) therapy in previously treated patients with chronic lymphocytic leukemia. *Ann Oncol.* 1996;7:373–379

44. Hiddemann W, Rottmann R, Wörmann B, Thiel A, Essink M, Ottensmeier C, Freund M, Büchner T, van de Loo J. Treatment of advanced chronic lymphocytic leukemia by fludarabine. Results of a clinical phase II study. *Ann Hematol.* 1991;63:1–4

45. Rondelli D, Lauria F, Zinzani PL, Raspadori D, Ventura MA, Galieni P, Birtolo S, Forconi F, Algeri R, Tura S. 2-Chlorodeoxyadenosine in the treatment of relapsed/refractory chronic lymphoproliferative disorders. *Eur J Haematol.* 1997;58:46–50

46. Rummel MJ, Kafer G, Pfreundschuh M, Jager E, Reinhardt U, Mitrou PS, Hoelzer D, Bergmann L. Fludarabine and epirubicin in the treatment of chronic lymphocytic leukaemia: a German multicenter phase II study. *Ann Oncol.* 1999;10:183–188

47. Spriano M, Clavio M, Carrara P, Canepa L, Miglino M, Pierri I, Celesti L, Rossi E, Vimercati R, Bruni R, *et al.* Fludarabine in untreated and previously treated B-CLL patients: a report on efficacy and toxicity. *Haematologica.* 1994;79:218–224

48. Sorensen JM, Vena DA, Fallavollita A, Chun HG, Cheson BD. Treatment of refractory chronic lymphocytic leukemia with fludarabine phosphate via the group C protocol mechanism of the National Cancer Institute: five-year follow-up report. *J Clin Oncol.* 1997;15:458–465

49. Saven A, Lemon RH, Kosty M, Beutler E, Piro LD. 2-Chlorodeoxyadenosine activity in patients with untreated chronic lymphocytic leukemia. *J Clin Oncol.* 1995;13:570–574

50. Rai KR, Peterson BL, Appelbaum FR, Kolitz J, Elias L, Shepherd L, Hines J, Threatte GA, Larson RA, Cheson BD, Schiffer CA. Fludarabine compared with chlorambucil as primary therapy for chronic lymphocytic leukemia. *N Engl J Med.* 2000;343:1750–1757

51. Tefferi A, Levitt R, Li CY, Schroeder G, Tschetter LK, Michalak JC, Krook JE, Witzig TE. Phase II study of 2-chlorodeoxyadenosine in combination with chlorambucil in previously untreated B-cell chronic lymphocytic leukemia. *Am J Clin Oncol.* 1999;22:509–516

52. Clavio M, Miglino M, Spriano M, Pietrasanta D, Vallebella E, Celesti L, Canepa L, Pierri I, Cavaliere M, Ballerini F, Beltrami G, Rossi E, Vimercati R, Bruni R, Congiu M, Nati S, Damasio E, Santini G, Gobbi M. First line fludarabine treatment of symptomatic chronic lymphoproliferative diseases: clinical results and molecular analysis of minimal residual disease. *Eur J Haematol.* 1998;61:197–203

53. Hocepied AM, Falkson CI, Falkson G. A phase II trial of fludarabine in patients with previously treated chronic lymphocytic leukaemia. *S Afr Med J.* 1996;86:549–550

54. Pillay GS, Wood L, Jacobs P. Fludarabine monophosphate as salvage for refractory chronic lymphocytic leukaemia. *S Afr Med J.* 1996;86:949–951

55. The French Cooperative Group on CLL. Randomized comparison of fludarabine, CAP and CHOP in 696 previously untreated patients. *Hematol Cell Ther.* 1997;39:S58–S59

56. Stelitano C, Morabito F, Kropp MG, Callea V, Iuliano F, Oriana V, Levato D, Nobile F, Molica S, Brugiatelli M. Fludarabine treatment in B-cell chronic lymphocytic leukemia: response, toxicity and survival analysis in 47 cases. *Haematologica.* 1999;84:317–323

57. McLaughlin P, Robertson LE, Keating MJ. Fludarabine phosphate in lymphoma: an important new therapeutic agent. *Cancer Treat Res.* 1996;85:3–14

58. Emmanouilides C, Rosen P, Rasti S, Territo M, Kunkel L. Treatment of indolent lymphoma with fludarabine/mitoxantrone combination: a phase II trial. *Hematol Oncol.* 1998;16:107–116

59. Magnac C, Sutton L, Cazin B, Laurent C, Binet JL, Merle-Beral H, Dighiero G, Maloum K. Detection of minimal residual disease in B chronic lymphocytic leukemia (CLL). *Hematol Cell Ther.* 1999;41:13–18

3

Monoclonal Antibodies in Cancer: The Development of Campath-1H

Since the Nobel prize-winning demonstration by Cesar Milstein that it is feasible to produce specific monoclonal antibodies (MAbs) using mouse hybridoma cell lines, one goal of their application has been to use this specificity as a tool to fight cancer. Hybridoma technology, in which fused cells in continuous culture produce rodent MAbs of the desired specificity, has now been supplemented by recombinant technology allowing MAbs tailored for particular applications to be produced from bacteriophage libraries. Chimeric MAbs, in which variable domains from rodent species are linked to constant domains from human immunoglobulins, have also been generated. This has gone a long way to overcoming one major problem encountered in the first clinical trials: the existence of a human antiglobulin response mounted against the foreign elements of the MAb, frequently found to limit the duration of effective therapy to 10 days[1].

Monoclonal antibodies directed against antigens found on the surface of the cancer cell can be used to directly modulate cell metabolism and to promote tumor lysis by immune effector cells and activation of complement. This innovative approach to cancer therapy is of particular significance as a method of treating tumors which are unresponsive or have become refractory to other methods of treatment, as is frequently the case with low-grade lymphomas, such as follicular non-Hodgkin's lymphoma, or B-CLL[2].

The first such MAb to gain FDA approval, in 1997, and so usher in this new type of tumor treatment, was rituximab. This is a chimeric anti-CD20 antibody which targets late pre-B-cells and differentiated B-cells, and has considerable effect in relapsing follicular NHL[3,4]. There are now a number of MAbs in development for NHL and associated disorders, shown in Table 1.

Table 1. Monoclonal antibodies in development for treatment of NHL/CLL

Antibody	Special features	Stage (Disease: NHL unless otherwise noted)	Target
Campath-1H	Unconjugated, anti B- and T-cell	Phase II Fast-track (B-CLL)	CD52
Rituximab (Rituxan)	Chimeric. Also used in conjunction with chemotherapy	Phase I/II/III Approved	CD20
Tositumab (Bexxar)	Linked to iodine-131 Synergy with fludarabine	Phase II	CD20
Ibritumomab tuixetan (Zevalin)	Linked to yttrium-90	Phase III (NHL/CLL)	D20
HulD10	Depletes B-cells, primarily by apoptosis	Phase I	HLA-DR-variant
Apratuzumab (hLL2)	Unconjugated, humanized	Phase I	CD22
CLB-CD19	Used in conjunction with IL-2	Phase I	CD19
LMB-2	Linked to immunotoxin	Phase II	CD25-receptor
BL22	Linked to immunotoxin	Phase I	CD22
HuM291	Success in psoriasis, now in phase I for NHL	Phase I (NHL)	CD3
HeFi-1	Active against Reed Sternberg cells in NHL	Phase I	CD20
VH4-34	Lyses B-cells by pore formation	Pre-clinical development	VH gene
CTLA4-Ig	Blocks T-cell co-stimulation, promotes engraftment	Pre-clinical development	B7/CD28
Anti-CTLA-4	Stimulates normal immune response	Pre-clinical development	B7/CD28

The Campath series of antibodies, directed against CD52, have considerable potential in both B- and T-cell malignancies and have already been used to purge T-cells prior to bone marrow transplantation to reduce the incidence of graft-versus-host disease. Being strongly lytic *in vivo* they can be used directly without the need to link to a radiolabel or immunotoxin to accentuate cell death. After early work using rodent IgG and IgM isotypes, the humanized form, Campath-1H has been generated by inserting rodent hypervariable sequences into a human framework in order to maximize its activity and minimize unwanted immunogenicity. This was the first antibody to be humanized and is now approved for refractory B-CLL, and in advanced disease for which other treatments have failed, it offers new hope.

The route to Campath-1H

The Campath-1 antibodies were first produced by a research team led by Professor Herman Waldmann in the Department of Pathology at Cambridge, UK. Their research effort focused upon developing therapeutic MAbs capable of cell killing using natural effector mechanisms, without a need for the antibody to be conjugated to a radiolabel or toxin (Figure 1). These antibodies were also selected because of their broad reactivity with normal and malignant human cells due to the nature and distribution of the antigen recognized. This antigen, designated CD52 by the Fourth International Workshop on Human Leukocyte Differentiation Antigens in 1989, has many of the features of a good candidate target also shown in Table 2, such as abundance on malignant cells, and cell surface expression which is not modulated during the cell cycle, or internalized in response to ligand binding[4-6].

Table 2. Desirable characteristics[4-6]

CD52		Campath series	
• Abundant on malignant cells	+++	• Promote complement-mediated lysis	++
• No variant or mutated antigens	+	• Promote tumor lysis by effector cells	+++
• Not internalized in response to antibody binding	+		
• Not shed or secreted in soluble form	+		

CD52 is expressed at high density (approximately 5×10^5 molecules per cell) on most mature normal and malignant lymphocytes but not on hematopoietic stem cells[5]. It is the shortest cell surface protein characterized to date, and, as shown in Figure 1, consists of 12 amino acids and a large, complex N-linked oligosaccharide, coupled to the membrane through an ethanolamine linkage to a glycosylphosphatidylinositol (GPI) anchor[6,7]. Such GPI-linked proteins are found in clusters on the cell surface, as shown schematically in Figure 1.

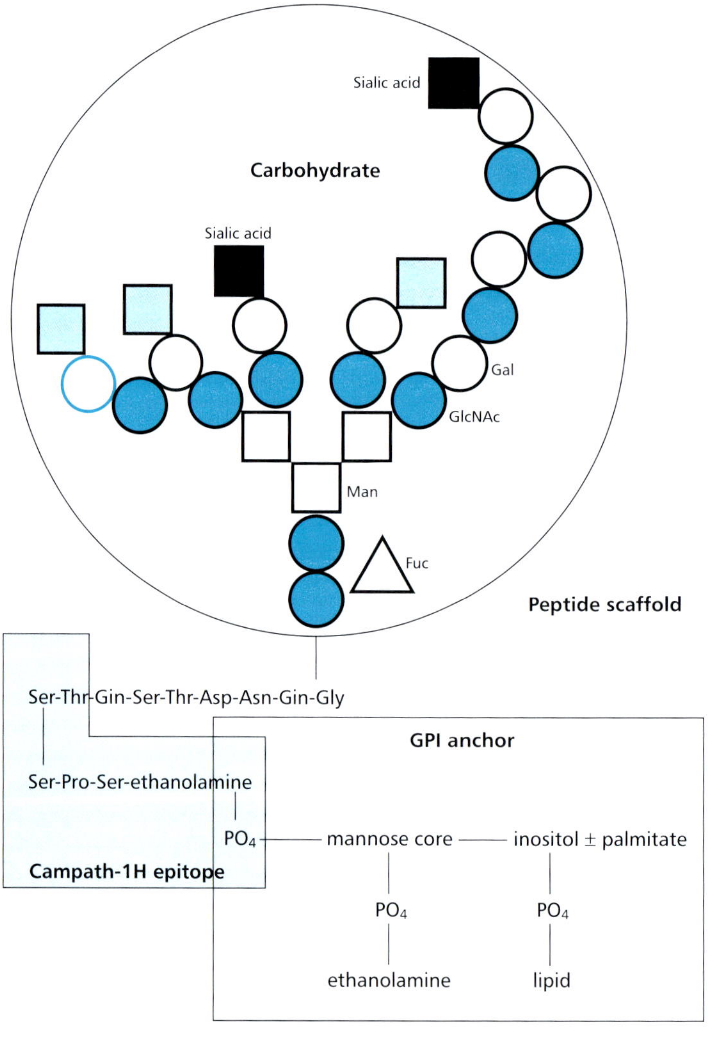

Figure 1. CD52 peptide

Reproduced with kind permission from Hale *et al*[6].

A variant, altered at the sugar moiety and at the membrane anchor[8], but with the same Campath-1H-binding epitope is found in epithelial cells of the male reproductive tract, particularly the epididymis[9]. This is shed into the seminal fluid where it is acquired by sperm[10]. It is present on the tail end of mature, highly motile spermatozoa[11] and binding Campath antibodies results in sperm agglutination[12,13]. Although sperm-specific CD52 antibodies have been proposed as a contraceptive, the small amounts of Campath able to reach the reproductive tract following systemic administration are likely to be too low to impair fertility.

The quantitative expression of CD52 on the malignant cell may correlate with the response to Campath treatment *in vivo*[14]. Binding of the antibody can, in principle, trigger cell death by three different mechanisms: complement activation, antibody-dependent cellular cytotoxicity (ADCC) and apoptosis. Most evidence points to cell death being ADCC-related, with cell killing able to occur via effector cells and via killing of antibody-coated lymphocytes by conventional phagocytosis and destruction in macrophages.

Complement-mediated cell lysis

The complement system consists of a set of up to 20 serum proteins that form a controlled cascade rapidly amplifying the production of activated molecules, as shown in Figure 2. The complete sequence occurs on the surface of the cell and is triggered by complement C1 recognition of a single IgM molecule or two clustered IgG molecules. After C1 binds to the clustered IgG, complement proteins C2 and C4 rapidly amplify the response. One molecule of activated C2aC4b (also known as C3 convertase) can cleave many molecules of C3. C3 splits into the anaphylotoxin C3a, and C3b, which triggers opsonization (enhancement of phagocytosis subsequent to binding of C3b to specific receptors on the macrophage surface) and also binds into a trimolecular complex with C3 convertase able to cleave C5 in the next step in the cascade. The resulting C5a has the most potent chemotactic and anaphylactic activity of any chemical mediator, while the other product, C5b, binds to the cell surface where it reacts with the remaining complement molecules, C6, 7, 8, and 9, to produce a multimolecular complex that can insert into the cell membrane, forming a channel through which the cytoplasm can be expelled.

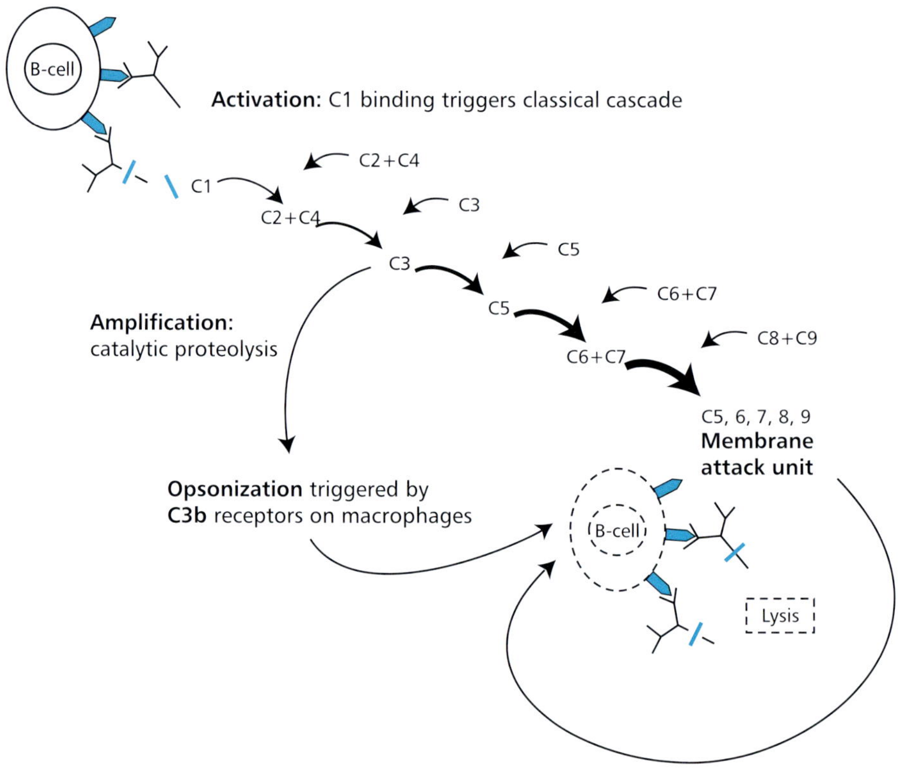

Figure 2. Complement-mediated cell lysis

Antibody-dependent cellular cytotoxicity

Antibody-dependent cellular cytotoxicity (ADCC) and its potential effector cells are shown in Figure 3. Immune effector cells which express Fc receptors[15] are capable of lysing tumors after binding to the Fc site. Levels of Fc receptor expression are under complex control by cytokines. Potential effector cells include neutrophils, macrophages, eosinophils and natural killer (NK) cells. NK cells, also known as large granular lymphocytes, which are a part of the non-adaptive immune system, are probably the most important mediators of ADCC[16]. ADCC is a very efficient way of lysing target cells because it requires significantly less antibody than complement-mediated lysis.

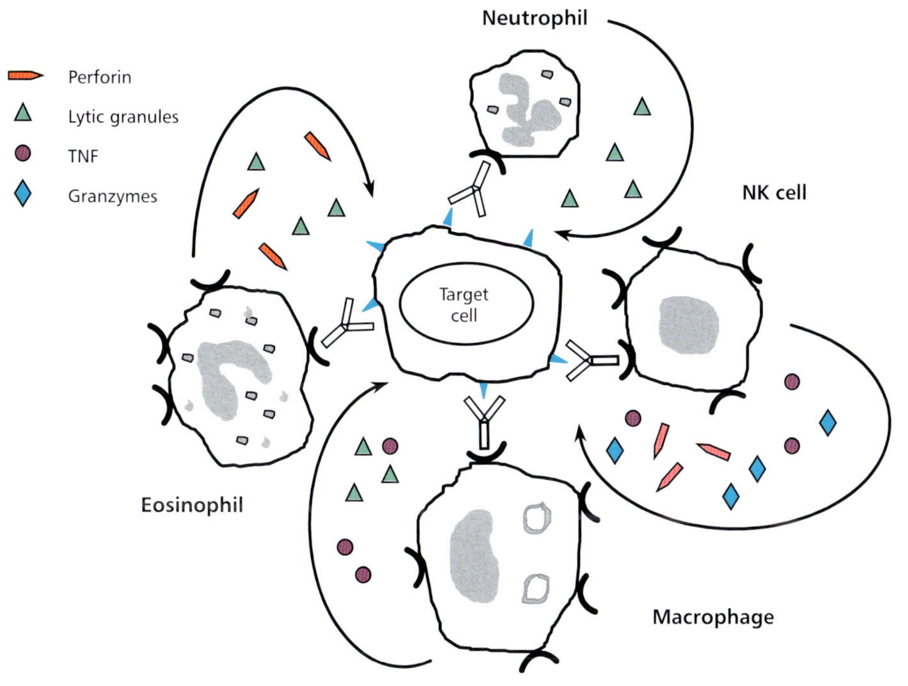

Figure 3. Antibody-dependent cellular cytotoxicity

The lytic mechanisms have been proposed to consist of polarized secretions of granule-stored molecules, occurring on effector-target cell contact. By electron microscopy, membrane deposited, pore-like lesions are detected on the target cell membrane during cytolysis. Further purification of proteins stored in these granules led to the discovery of a membranolytic protein named perforin which is capable of polymerizing into pore-like structures. In addition to this cytolytic protein, a set of serine esterases are produced, as well as lysosomal enzymes and proteoglycans, whose functions are not yet clearly defined[17]. Macrophages and NK cells can also act by releasing tumor necrosis factor alpha (TNF-α), and proteolytic enzymes (granzymes) which cleave and activate key molecules in target cells. Because of their ability to activate caspases and post-caspase enzymes in apoptotic cascades, granzymes have been implicated in apoptotic cell death as well as in lytic necrosis[18,19]. Allowing granzymes and other lytic enzymes access to the target cell may be an important role for perforin, in addition to its ability to punch holes in the cell membrane for cytoplasm expulsion, as described for the membrane attack complex after complement activation.

The relative importance of each of these effector cells and their varied functions are not yet known, but studies have shown that ADCC can be enhanced by use of specific cytokines. G-CSF and GM-CSF[20] can be used after application of therapeutic MAbs[21].

Apoptosis

Another possible method of cell death after Campath binding is by apoptosis (Figure 4). Much *in vitro* work has been carried out to explore induction of apoptosis by Campath antibodies, and while there is some evidence that this occurs, this work has not as yet been confirmed by *in vivo* studies.

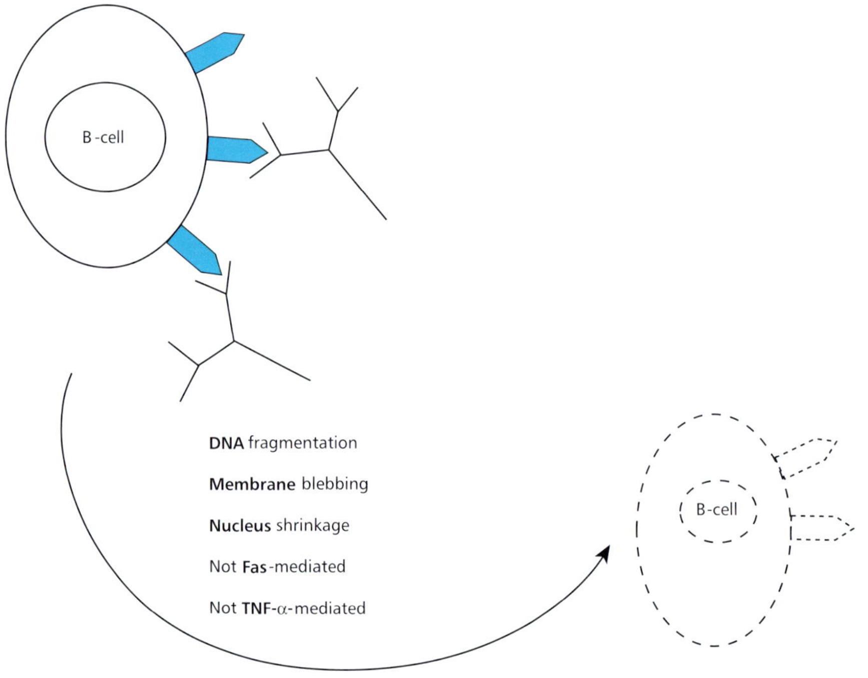

Figure 4. Apoptotic cell death

Antibodies against GPI molecules, when cross-linked by a secondary anti-immunoglobulin *in vitro*, produce slow and incomplete growth inhibition of B-cells, which trigger internal cell signals shown to result in cell accumulation at the G_0/G_1 boundary and apoptotic cell death in the B-cell line Wien133[22,23]. In the case of the Campath series, apoptotic signalling does not rely upon Fas ligand binding at the cell membrane (see Chapter 1). Although Campath antibodies can stimulate T-cell proliferation *in vitro,* the significance of this to the destructive effect *in vivo* remains unclear. Apoptotic cell death is not reliant on CD52 expression at high density on the cell surface but may be heavily influenced by the presence of an activated immune system. As previously mentioned, there may be overlap between apoptotic cell death and ADCC, since granzymes released after binding of effector cells to Fc receptors can activate caspases as shown in Figure 5. The caspase dependence of cytoplasmic changes in response to granzymes has been examined by work using Jurkat cells in culture[19]. This study indicated that when caspases are inhibited, lysis can still occur, but nuclear fragmentation is prevented, indicating that in addition to activation of caspases, granzymes can directly trigger a postcaspase cytoplasmic death pathway. In contrast, Fas-ligand-induced apoptosis was completely blocked by *in vitro* caspase inhibition, preventing both lysis and nuclear fragmentation.

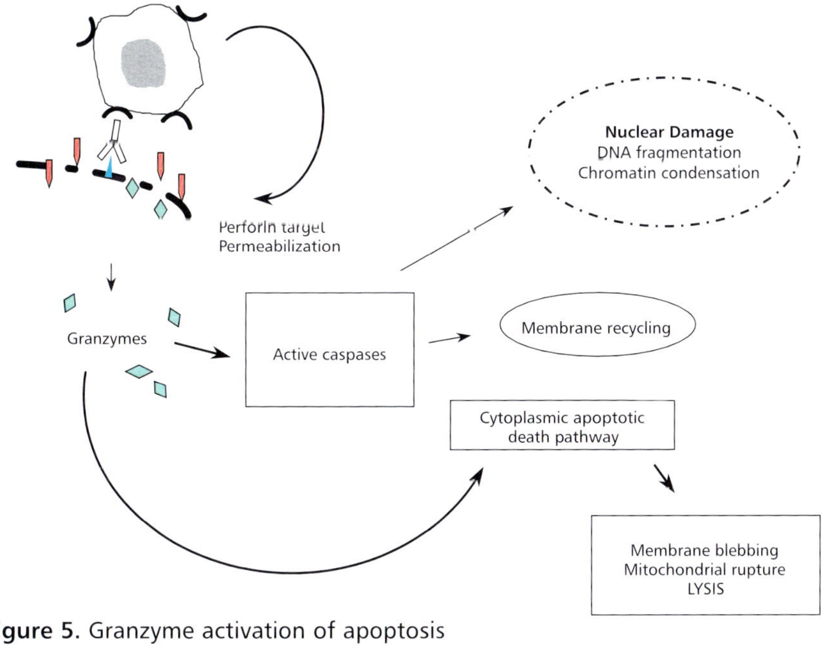

Figure 5. Granzyme activation of apoptosis

Campath-1H action *in vivo*

While the contributions of these three mechanisms of cell killing are not precisely defined, it seems likely that ADCC plays the largest role *in vivo*. The presence of site-specific effector cells may explain the longer term efficacy of Campath-1H-induced killing of lymphocytes in marrow and lymph node and transient effects on cells in peripheral blood.

Isotypes of Campath

Early work using rodent isotypes of Campath showed that different isotypes varied in their ability to trigger these mechanisms of cell killing. All rat IgM and IgG versions of Campath were lytic with human complement, producing transient depletion in blood lymphocytes, but only the rat IgGb form was active in ADCC and produced effects on tumor mass or bone marrow. This demonstrated the importance of the Fc interaction for effective clearance of target cells *in vivo*. Of human IgG isotypes, IgG_1 and IgG_3 are most effective for both complement-mediated lysis and ADCC[24–26]. These factors were taken into account when the Campath-1H antibody was produced by building rat antigen-binding sites, into a human antibody framework to produce the Campath-1H IgG shown in Figures 6 and 7.

The production of chimeric molecules, splicing hypervariable regions from one species to constant regions from another, has been used for some antibodies such as Rituxan, this may still result in molecules which provoke an immune response[27]. In order to minimize this risk, Campath-1H was humanized, being the first antibody to undergo this process, in which short rodent sequence fragments responsible for antigen recognition were embedded into an entirely human IgG framework[28].

The antigen-binding site in Campath-1H was derived from a rat IgG_{2a} where the hypervariable regions were identified at the sequence level. These three regions of the heavy chain were synthesized as large oligonucleotides and mounted into human variable regions of both light (REI sequence)[29] and heavy (NEW sequence)[30] human IgG chains expressed from plasmid constructs under the control of the heavy chain promotor. Figure 6 shows how the different domains were assembled into the final molecule in a three-step process which allowed partly humanized antibodies to be checked for functional activity (by both complement lysis and by direct binding) at each stage.

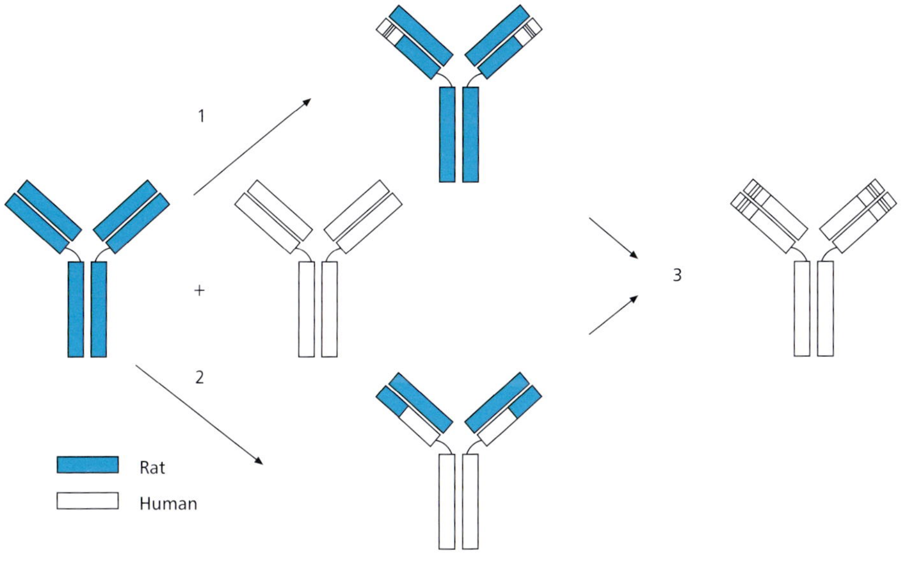

Figure 6. Reshaping of Campath-1H
Adapted from Riechmann *et al*[28].

In stage 1, the reshaped human/rat heavy chain variable domain was attached to constant domains of the rat isotype IgG_{2b}, shown in black, and transfected into a variant hybridoma cell line lacking the ability to produce its own heavy chain. The reshaped molecule bound antigen more weakly than the original IgG_{2a}, expressed in the same way, due to a variation in the human framework sequence which altered stacking of one hypervariable loop of the antigen-binding region. A single amino acid change at position 27 from serine to phenylalanine was introduced and found to fully restore antigen-binding activity. This re-shaped variable region was therefore suitable to be inserted into a fully human framework.

In stage two, the rat heavy variable region was attached to constant domains of human isotypes IgG_{1-4}, and expressed in the same hybridoma. Assessment of activity showed that IgG_4 proved to be completely unable to function in complement lysis of human lymphocytes. IgG_3 was weakly lytic, IgG_2 was more active but still less strongly lytic than the original rat IgG_{2b}, and only human IgG_1 proved to be comparable in strength of activity.

In stage three, the re-shaped heavy chain, and the re-shaped light chain were attached to the human IgG_1 isotype constant regions. The two clones were co-transfected into a non-secreting rat myeloma cell line.

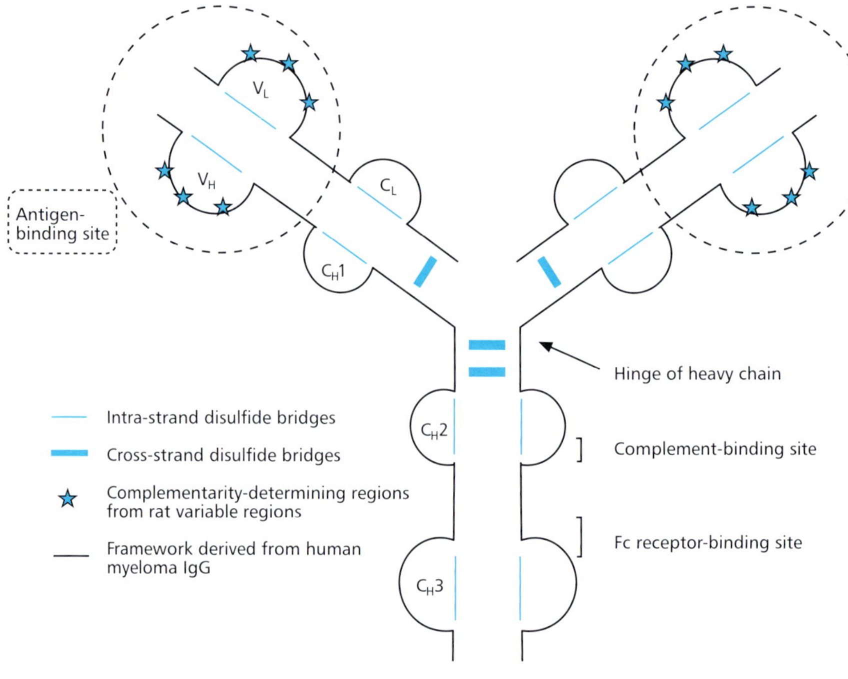

Figure 7. Humanized Campath IgG

The resultant antibody bound tightly to CD52 and proved as effective as rat IgG_{2b} in complement lysis. It was more effective in cell-mediated lysis than the rat antibody from which the variable regions were derived. Like Campath-1G, the humanized version of Campath remains unable to deplete hematopoietic stem cells[5].

The development of this antibody with *in vivo* potency and reduced immunogenicity allowed more extensive studies on its action on the immune system to be carried out, and paved the way for key clinical studies. Its decreased immunogenicity was of particular significance in allowing treatment of chronic disorders involving aberrant T-cell populations, such as rheumatoid arthritis (RA)[31-33] and multiple sclerosis (MS)[34,35], which may require repeated cycles of treatment. Other auto-immune disorders in which it has provided effective long-term benefit are systemic vasculitis[36] and refractory Wegener's granulomatosis[37,38].

The effects of Campath-1H *in vivo*

The CD52 antigen is expressed on virtually all lymphocytes including T- and B-cells, on NK cells, eosinophils and macrophages but is absent from erythrocytes, platelets and bone marrow progenitor cells[39,40]. The fact that Campath-1H does not deplete stem cells means that it can be used to rapidly purge mature malignant cells from blood and marrow without permanent immunodepletion since the stem cell population remains intact and capable of replenishing functional mature B- and T-cells.

Campath-1H exerts a strong first-dose reaction, associated with the release of inflammatory cytokines including TNF-α, IL-6/IL-10 and IFN-γ[41,42]. Schedules of increasing dosage of Campath-1H, and the introduction of concomitant medication are used to moderate the strength of this reaction, with its associated malaise, hypotension, fever, rigors and chills. Nausea and vomiting can also result, but in a relatively mild form which bears little resemblance to the side-effects of chemotherapy with alkylating agents such as chlorambucil. These acute reactions are usually seen within the first week of therapy after which symptoms moderate.

After therapy with large doses of Campath 1H, there is profound lymphopenia; CD16+ (NK cells) are the first to recover, since they are largely spared by Campath-1H[32], achieving pre-treatment levels within 40 days; CD8+ cells recover by 6 months, but CD4+ cells take longer and in many patients remain subnormal at 4 years[31], especially where previous lympholytic drugs have been used in treatment.

Individuals with late-stage disease may already be immunosuppressed, either due to progression or as a result of previous treatments. However, the clinical consequences of peripheral blood CD4+ depletion are not clear-cut, and patients who do not appear to show an increased risk of infection despite low CD4+ counts in the blood may have adequate CD4+ counts in lymph nodes.

The restoration of lymphocyte counts is sometimes accompanied by the emergence of CD52-negative subclones which fail to express GPI-linked proteins[43–45].

In an early study in heavily pre-treated B-CLL cases, seven patients with disease refractory to fludarabine were treated with Campath-1H[46]. A subcutaneous route of administration was used, in order to minimize first-dose effects. Durable responses were seen in four patients, with two of three patients after partial response (PR) being successfully retreated with Campath-1H and achieving a second (PR). Many of these patients, however, experienced opportunistic infections, primarily cytomegalovirus reactivation, likely to be related to immunodepletion due to prior treatment regimens. Similarly, in a phase II study of relapsed or refractory B-CLL, major responses were seen in 43% of 29 patients accompanied by opportunistic infections or bacterial septicemia[47]. A phase II trial of heavily pre-treated low-grade NHL showed comparable results; 50% of 50 patients responded, with nine patients developing opportunistic infections and nine bacterial septicemia[48].

In order for the promise of Campath-1H to be fulfilled in B-CLL, treatment regimens have been adapted to reduce susceptibility to opportunistic infection. PhaseI/II dose-ranging trials were designed and carried out, using dosing regimens of once weekly, three times a week and five times a week, with patients stratified by disease type and given the same dose, as shown in Table 3.

Table 3. Dose-ranging trial designs

Protocol	Patients	Dosing regimen	Assigned cohort unit dose (mg) and patient number (*n*)											
			1		2		3		4		5		6	
			mg	*n*	mg	*n*	mg	*n*	mg	*n*	mg	*n*	mg	*n*
002	71	Once a week	7.5	13	24	16	75	22	240	20	—	—	—	—
003	36	Five times a week	0.5	5	5.0	5	5.0	8	5.0	7	5.0	7	50	4
001	68	Three times a week	2.5	12	8.0	12	25	14	80	30	—	—	—	—

With repeated dosing it was found that patients developed tolerance to first-dose effects, whereas with once-weekly treatment they often experienced the same intensity of adverse reactions with each infusion. The results indicated that a dose of at least 25 mg but less than 80 mg given three times a week provided the best benefit to risk ratio. They also indicated that dose escalation would minimize initial adverse reactions. These dose-ranging trials did not include compulsory prophylaxis.

Campath-1H is now being used in a dose escalation regimen with pre-medication for amelioration of cytokine-mediated symptoms and as prophylaxis for infection.

Recommended premedications and prophylaxis are shown in Table 4.

Table 4. Premedications (A) and prophylaxis (B) to optimize Campath-1H response

	A	
Systemic symptoms	**Pre-medication**	**Administration**
Rigors/chills	50 mg i.v. diphenylhydramine 500–650 mg acetaminophen meperidine	1 hour prior to Campath administration 30 min prior to Campath administration
Tumor lysis syndrome	allopurinol $NaHCO_3$ fluids	*ADI
Rash	H_1-blockers	ADI
Hypotension	H_2-blockers e.g. cimetidine, famotidine, ranitidine	ADI
Nausea/ vomiting	anti-emetics, e.g. serotonin antagonists, antihistamines, or pheothiazines	ADI
	B	
Opportunistic infections	**Prophylactic**	**Administration**
Pneumocystis	trimethoprim/sulfamethazole or dapsone or pentamidine	Optional
Herpes	acyclovir or famcyclovir	Optional
Aspergillus	itraconazole Optional	
Candida	fluconazole Optional	

*ADI, At the discretion of the investigator

The dose-escalation regimen currently recommended is to treat patients initially with intravenous Campath-1H at 3 mg during a 2-hour infusion period, up to five times a week until this dose is tolerated without acute infusion-related effects. Several infusions at the lower dose may be needed, then the dose can be rapidly escalated through 10 mg infusions to 30 mg and continued three times weekly for a period of 8 weeks to a maximum of 12 weeks. In the event of a temporary loss of venous access the dose can be administered in the form of subcutaneous injection in divided doses of no more than 1 ml per injection. Ideally, on day 1 patients will receive 3 mg, on day 2, 10 mg and on day 3, 30 mg. However, several treatments at the lower doses may be necessary. Premedications with diphenylhydramine and acetaminophen are given 30 minutes prior to first dose, at each dose-escalation and thereafter as clinically indicated.

In an initial report of nine patients with previously untreated, progressive B-CLL, minimal first-dose effects of fever and rigor were apparent in all but one patient, followed by major and prolonged disease remission, with three patients achieving complete remission and five patients a partial response [49].

Results showing efficacy in a small number of cases, with good responses in blood and bone marrow and lesser responses in reduction of bulky nodal disease, supported the need for trials of Campath-1H to be undertaken in order to demonstrate its utility in patients with refractory disease. The results of three phase II trials, including the pivotal trial 211, are described in detail in Chapter 4.

Reference List

1. Weiner LM. Monoclonal antibody therapy of cancer. *Semin Oncology*. 1999;26:43–51
2. Alpaugh K, von Mehren, M. Monoclonal antibodies in cancer treatment: a review of recent progress. *BioDrugs*. 1999;12:209–236
3. Winkler U, Jensen M, Manzke O, Schulz H, Diehl V, Engert A. Cytokine-release syndrome in patients with B-cell chronic lymphocytic leukemia and high lymphocyte counts after treatment with an anti-CD20 monoclonal antibody (rituximab, IDEC-C2B8). *Blood*. 1999;94:2217–2224
4. Maloney DG. Advances in immunotherapy of hematologic malignancies. *Curr Opin Hematol*. 1998;5:237–243
5. Gilleece MH, Dexter TM. Effect of Campath-1H antibody on human hematopoietic progenitors *in vitro*. *Blood*. 1993;82:807–812
6. Hale G. Synthetic peptide mimotope of the CAMPATH-1 (CD52) antigen, a small glycosylphosphatidylinositol-anchored glycoprotein. *Immunotechnology*. 1995;1:175–187
7. Treumann A, Lifely MR, Schneider P, Ferguson MA. Primary structure of CD52. *J Biol Chem*. 1995;270:6088–6099
8. Schroter S, Derr P, Conradt HS, Nimtz M, Hale G, Kirchhoff C. Male-specific modification of human CD52. *J Biol Chem*. 1999;274:29862–29873
9. Hale G, Rye PD, Warford A, Lauder I, Brito-Babapulle A. The glycosylphosphatidylinositol-anchored lymphocyte antigen CDw52 is associated with the epididymal maturation of human spermatozoa. *J Reprod Immunol*. 1993;23:189–205
10. Kirchhoff C. CD52 is the 'major maturation-associated' sperm membrane antigen. *Mol Hum Reprod*. 1996;2:9–17
11. Focarelli R, Della Giovampaola C, Seraglia R, Brettoni C, Sabatini L, Pescaglini M, Rosati F. Biochemical and MALDI analysis of the human sperm antigen gp20, homologue of leukocyte CD52. *Biochem Biophys Res Commun*. 1999;258:639–643
12. Yeung CH, Schroter S, Wagenfeld A, Kirchhoff C, Kliesch S, Poser D, Weinbauer GF, Nieschlag E, Cooper TG. Interaction of the human epididymal protein CD52 (HE5) with epididymal spermatozoa from men and cynomolgus monkeys. *Mol Reprod Dev*. 1997; 48:267–275
13. Yeung CH, Cooper TG, Nieschlag E. Human epididymal secreted protein CD52 on ejaculated spermatozoa: correlations with semen characteristics and the effect of its antibody. *Mol Hum Reprod*. 1997;3:1045–1051
14. Ginaldi L, De Martinis M, Matutes E, Farahat N, Morilla R, Dyer MJ, Catovsky D. Levels of expression of CD52 in normal and leukemic B and T cells: correlation with *in vivo* therapeutic responses to Campath-1H. *Leuk Res*. 1998;22:185–191
15. van de Winkel JG, Capel PJ. Human IgG Fc receptor heterogeneity: molecular aspects and clinical implications. *Immunol Today*. 1993;14:215–221
16. Rees RC. MHC restricted and non-restricted killer lymphocytes. *Blood Rev*. 1990;4:204–210
17. Lowin B, Krahenbuhl O, Muller C, Dupuis M, Tschopp J. Perforin and its role in T lymphocyte-mediated cytolysis. *Experientia*. 1992;48:911–920
18. Henkart PA, Williams MS, Zacharchuk CM, Sarin A. Do CTL kill target cells by inducing apoptosis? *Semin Immunol*. 1997;9:135–144
19. Sarin A, Haddad EK, Henkart PA. Caspase dependence of target cell damage induced by cytotoxic lymphocytes. *J Immunol*. 1998;161:2810–2816

20. Cairo MS, VandeVen C, Toy C, Mauss D, Sheikh K, Kommareddy S, Modanlou H. Lymphokines: enhancement by granulocyte-macrophage and granulocyte colony-stimulating factors of neonatal myeloid kinetics and functional activation of polymorphonuclear leukocytes. *Rev Infect Dis.* 1990;12 Suppl 4:S492–S497

21. Valerius T, Elsasser D, Repp R, Van de Winkel JG, Gramatzki M, Glennie M. HLA class II antibodies recruit G-CSF activated neutrophils for treatment of B cell malignancies. *Leuk Lymphoma.* 1997;26:261–269

22. Rowan WC, Hale G, Tite JP, Brett SJ. Cross-linking of the CAMPATH-1 antigen (CD52) triggers activation of normal human T lymphocytes. *Int Immunol.* 1995;7:69–77

23. Rowan W, Tite J, Topley P, Brett SJ. Cross-linking of the CAMPATH-1 antigen (CD52) mediates growth inhibition in human B- and T-lymphoma cell lines, and subsequent emergence of CD52-deficient cells. *Immunology.* 1998;95:427–436

24. Bruggemann M, Williams GT, Bindon CI, Clark MR, Walker MR, Jefferis R, Waldmann H, Neuberger MS. Comparison of the effector functions of human immunoglobulins using a matched set of chimeric antibodies. *J Exp Med.* 1987;166:1351–1361

25. Greenwood J, Clark M, Waldmann H. Structural motifs involved in human IgG antibody effector functions. *Eur J Immunol.* 1993;23:1098–1104

26. Greenwood J, Gorman SD, Routledge EG, Lloyd IS, Waldmann H. Engineering multiple-domain forms of the therapeutic antibody CAMPATH-1H: effects on complement lysis. *Ther Immunol.* 1994;1:247–255

27. Bruggemann M, Winter G, Waldmann H, Neuberger MS. The immunogenicity of chimeric antibodies. *J Exp Med.* 1989;170:2153–2157

28. Riechmann L, Clark M, Waldmann H, Winter G. Reshaping human antibodies for therapy. *Nature.* 1988;332:323–327

29. Saul FA, Amzel LM, Poljak RJ. Preliminary refinement and structural analysis of the Fab fragment from human immunoglobulin new at 2.0 A resolution. *J Biol Chem.* 1978;253: 585–597

30. Epp O, Colman P, Fehlhammer H, Bode W, Schiffer M, Huber R, Palm W. Crystal and molecular structure of a dimer composed of the variable portions of the Bence-Jones protein REI. *Eur J Biochem.* 1974;45:513–524

31. Isaacs JD, Watts RA, Hazleman BL, Hale G, Keogan MT, Cobbold SP, Waldmann H. Humanised monoclonal antibody therapy for rheumatoid arthritis. *Lancet.* 1992;340:748–752

32. Watts RA, Isaacs JD, Hale G, Hazleman BL, Waldmann H. CAMPATH-1H in inflammatory arthritis. *Clin Exp Rheumatol.* 1993;11 Suppl 8:S165–S167

33. Isaacs JD, Manna VK, Rapson N, Bulpitt KJ, Hazleman BL, Matteson EL, St. Clair EW, Schnitzer TJ, Johnston JM. CAMPATH-1H in rheumatoid arthritis—an intravenous dose-ranging study. *Br J Rheumatol.* 1996;35:231–240

34. Moreau T, Coles A, Wing M, Thorpe J, Miller D, Moseley I, Issacs J, Hale G, Clayton D, Scolding N, Waldmann H, Compston A. CAMPATH-IH in multiple sclerosis. *Mult Scler.* 1996;1:357–365

35. Coles AJ, Wing MG, Molyneux P, Paolillo A, Davie CM, Hale G, Miller D, Waldmann H, Compston A. Monoclonal antibody treatment exposes three mechanisms underlying the clinical course of multiple sclerosis. *Ann Neurol.* 1999;46:296–304

36. Lockwood CM, Thiru S, Isaacs JD, Hale G, Waldmann H. Long-term remission of intractable systemic vasculitis with monoclonal antibody therapy. *Lancet.* 1993;341:1620–1622

37. Lockwood CM. Refractory Wegener's granulomatosis: a model for shorter immunotherapy of autoimmune diseases. *J R Coll Physicians Lond.* 1998;32:473–478

38. Lockwood CM, Thiru S, Stewart S, Hale G, Isaacs J, Wraight P, Elliott J, Waldmann H. Treatment of refractory Wegener's granulomatosis with humanized monoclonal antibodies [see comments]. *QJM.* 1996;89:903–912

39. Hale G, Bright S, Chumbley G, Hoang T, Metcalf D, Munro AJ, Waldmann H. Removal of T cells from bone marrow for transplantation: a monoclonal antilymphocyte antibody that fixes human complement. *Blood.* 1983;62:873–882

40. Hale G, Swirsky DM, Hayhoe FG, Waldmann H. Effects of monoclonal anti-lymphocyte antibodies *in vivo* in monkeys and humans. *Mol Biol Med.* 1983;1:321–334

41. Moreau T, Coles A, Wing M, Isaacs J, Hale G, Waldmann H, Compston A. Transient increase in symptoms associated with cytokine release in patients with multiple sclerosis. *Brain.* 1996;119(Pt 1):225–237

42. Wing MG, Moreau T, Greenwood J, Smith RM, Hale G, Isaacs J, Waldmann H, Lachmann PJ, Compston A. Mechanism of first-dose cytokine-release syndrome by CAMPATH 1-H: involvement of CD16 (FcgammaRIII) and CD11a/CD18 (LFA-1) on NK cells. *J Clin Invest.* 1996;98:2819–2826

43. Taylor VC, Sims M, Brett S, Field MC. Antibody selection against CD52 produces a paroxysmal nocturnal haemoglobinuria phenotype in human lymphocytes by a novel mechanism. *Biochem J.* 1997;322(Pt 3):919–925

44. Rawstron AC, Rollinson SJ, Richards S, Short MA, English A, Morgan GJ, Hale G, Hillmen P. The PNH phenotype cells that emerge in most patients after CAMPATH-1H therapy are present prior to treatment. *Br J Haematol.* 1999;107:148–153

45. Brett SJ, Baxter G, Cooper H, Rowan W, Regan T, Tite J, Rapson N. Emergence of CD52-, glycosylphosphatidylinositol-anchor-deficient lymphocytes in rheumatoid arthritis patients following Campath-1H treatment. *Int Immunol.* 1996;8:325–334

46. Bowen AL, Zomas A, Emmett E, Matutes E, Dyer MJ, Catovsky D. Subcutaneous CAMPATH-1H in fludarabine-resistant/relapsed chronic lymphocytic and B-prolymphocytic leukaemia. *Br J Haematol.* 1997;96:617–619

47. Osterborg A, Dyer MJ, Bunjes D, Pangalis GA, Bastion Y, Catovsky D, Mellstedt H. Phase II multicenter study of human CD52 antibody in previously treated chronic lymphocytic leukemia. European Study Group of CAMPATH-1H Treatment in Chronic Lymphocytic Leukemia. *J Clin Oncol.* 1997;15:1567–1574

48. Lundin J, Osterborg A, Brittinger G, Crowther D, Dombret H, Engert A, Epenetos A, Gisselbrecht C, Huhn D, Jaeger U, Thomas J, Marcus R, Nissen N, Poynton C, Rankin E, Stahel R, Uppenkamp M, Willemze R, Mellstedt H. CAMPATH-1H monoclonal antibody in therapy for previously treated low-grade non-Hodgkin's lymphomas: a phase II multicenter study. European Study Group of CAMPATH-1H Treatment in Low-Grade Non-Hodgkin's Lymphoma. *J Clin Oncol.* 1998;16:3257–3263

49. Osterborg A, Fassas AS, Anagnostopoulos A, Dyer MJ, Catovsky D, Mellstedt H. Humanized CD52 monoclonal antibody Campath-1H as first-line treatment in chronic lymphocytic leukaemia. *Br J Haematol.* 1996;93:151 153

Campath-1H in B-CLL: Remission of Refractory Disease

Campath-1H has now been used to treat patients with relapsed or refractory B-CLL in three Phase II clinical trials. While many clinical trials assessing chemotherapy for B-CLL exclude patients over a certain age, usually age 75 years[1-3], none of the Campath phase II trials, studies 005, 009, and 211, had an age cut-off point, in keeping with the pressing need for safe and efficacious therapy for patients with advanced, refractory B-CLL, many of whom are elderly.

The escalating dosage regimen used in studies 005 and 009 is shown in Figure 1. A lower initial dose was used in study 211 in which the starting dose of Campath-1H was 3 mg. Premedication used acetaminophen and antihistamines. In addition, an amendment in protocol 005 allowed doses to be administered by subcutaneous injection to selected patients. The main differences between the early studies, 005 and 009, and study 211 initiated later, were in the recommended prophylaxis, particularly with regard to the 2 months immediately after treatment. In studies 005 and 009, which had essentially identical protocols but were carried out in Europe and in the USA, respectively, prophylaxis for opportunistic infections was not routine at this time-point, and the observation that this was a period of vulnerability emphasized the need for precautions in subsequent protocols. In study 211, prophylactic clotrimazole and famcyclovir were used during and for 2 months after treatment was completed.

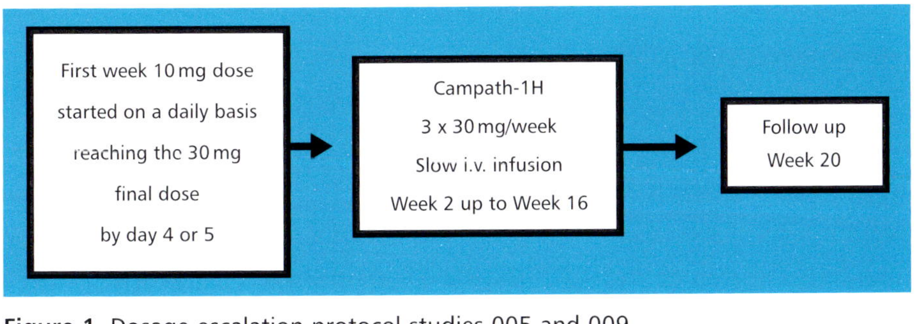

Figure 1. Dosage escalation protocol studies 005 and 009

In order to be eligible for either study 005, the European multi-center trial, or study 009, the American multi-center trial, B-CLL patients had to have disease-related symptoms, anemia and/or thrombocytopenia, bulky lymphadenopathy and/or splenomegaly that had caused compressive problems.

Of 29 B-CLL patients with previously treated disease enrolled in study 005, eight had relapsed after an initial response to chemotherapy and 21 were refractory to at least one alkylating agent-containing regimen[4]. Twelve patients completed the planned 12-week treatment period. Of the remaining 17 patients, ten were withdrawn early because of unresponsiveness, two rapidly achieved partial response and stabilized by 6 weeks, at which point treatment was terminated, one patient withdrew consent, and four were withdrawn because of serious infections.

Overall responses and response by site are shown in Table 1.

Table 1. Responses in previously treated patients[4] (NCI guidelines) Study 005

	CR		PR		SD		PD	
	%	*n*	%	*n*	%	*n*	%	*n*
Overall response (*n*=29)	4	1/29	38	11/29	41	12/29	17	5/29
Response by disease site								
Blood (*n*=29)*	97	28/29	3	1/29	—	—	—	—
Bone marrow (*n*=25)	36	9/25	16	4/25	36	9/25	12	3/25
Spleen (*n*=19)	32	6/19	26	5/19	42	8/19	—	—
Lymph node (*n*=28)	7	2/28	25	7/28	50	14/28	18	5/28

* Refers to resolution of lymphocytosis

Of the 12 responding patients, five achieved response after 6 weeks of treatment, and seven at week 12. Of the 21 chemotherapy refractory patients, nine responded to Campath-1H, and of the eight patients in relapse after initial treatment on trial entry, three responded to Campath-1H.

As shown in Table 1, malignant cells were completely purged from the blood in 28 patients within a median response period of 14 days (range 7–42), with the remaining patient showing a partial response by the end of treatment. Typically, after a 14-day lag time, Campath-1H cleared CLL cells from the blood until they were no longer detectable after 5 weeks of treatment. This was accompanied by an initial drop in platelet counts, subsequently replenished by regeneration from marrow stem cells with counts rising by week 7 of therapy. Platelet concentrations continued to increase gradually in responders and, even in patients who were thrombocytopenic at entry, reached normal levels (150×10^9/l) by week 12. Disease-related neutropenia was also alleviated in most responding patients in the course of treatment. Complete morphological remission was observed in nine patients, with four patients achieving partial marrow remission (more than 50% reduction in marrow infiltration). Four of these patients were monitored off-treatment for more than 2 years without additional progression.

Responses in the spleen were less dramatic than in blood or marrow, but in six of 19 patients, splenomegaly resolved completely, in five patients it resolved by >50% and in the remaining eight patients it remained unchanged. Enlarged lymph nodes disappeared in two of 28 patients, were reduced by >50% in seven patients, and progressed in five patients. Bulky disease at lymph nodes rather than the number of affected nodes was associated with poorer resolution of disease. The regression of enlarged lymph nodes usually required 8–12 weeks of therapy.

Additional results within the Study 005 trial have also demonstrated that Campath-1H can be used to facilitate a peripheral blood stem cell harvest for autologous transplantation[5]. Ten patients were treated at Leeds General Infirmary and Pinderfields General Hospital, Wakefield, UK, all refractory to conventional chemotherapy including fludarabine. The extent of residual disease in these patients was measured immunophenotypically using four-color flow cytometry. This is more sensitive than the NCI recommendations for complete response and partial response criteria, which rely upon resolution of lymphocytosis without assessment of residual disease in the form of any remaining malignant cells. Responses in cell counts after short (6-week) treatments, analyzed using this technique, which can detect one target cell against a background of 10,000 non-target cells, are shown in Table 2.

Table 2. Demonstration of response to Campath-1H by immunophenotyping

	Pre-Campath1H	Week 3	Week 6
CLL-blood ($\times 10^9$/l)	9.6 (range 0–85.7, *n*=8)	0 (range 0–0.007, *n*=8)	0 (range 0–0.027, *n*=6)
CLL-marrow (%)	56 (range 3–83, *n*=7)	5.5 (range 0–90, *n*=7)	0.8 (range 0–92, *n*=6)

Such immunophenotyping shows that responses can be achieved at the level of the malignant cell in both blood and marrow. As with other reports, the ability to achieve a complete remission was inversely related to the presence of bulky lymphadenopathy. All five patients who achieved complete response had no significant nodal disease, whereas the two patients with bulky disease only achieved PR. The last of these patients went into PR after just five doses of Campath-1H; his peripheral blood stem cells were then harvested for autografting, after CD34 enrichment of the harvested cells, and his lymphadenopathy entered regression subsequent to transplantation.

Another patient cohort analysis in which NCI criteria were supplemented by assessment of the disease at the cellular level using immunophenotyping was carried out at the Royal Marsden NHS Trust, London[6]. Campath-1H was used to treat six patients who had been treated to maximal response with fludarabine or deoxycoformycin (Table 3). Malignant cells were estimated using dual-color flow cytometry with directly labelled antibodies to tally cells co-expressing CD5 and CD19 (a sensitive marker for most cases of B-CLL). Campath-1H was administered at least 4 weeks after the last purine analogue treatment, and was given for 4–6 weeks or until repeat bone marrow aspirate and trephine biopsy showed no residual leukemic infiltration. Campath-1H successfully purged malignant cells from these patients in whom persistent leukemic infiltration had previously precluded bone marrow transplantation, allowing transplantation to be carried out (discussed further in Chapter 5).

Table 3. Response to Campath-1H in refractory patients[6]

	Previous therapy	Duration of Campath-1H therapy (weeks)	Bone marrow infiltration pre-Campath-1H	Bone marrow infiltration post-Campath-1H
1	Chlorambucil/ prednisolone, fludarabine	6	Aspirate: 37% Trephine: 30% CD5/CD19: 66%	Aspirate: CR Trephine: CR CD5/CD19: 1%
2	Chlorambucil/ prednisolone, CHOP, fludarabine	5	Aspirate: 69% Trephine: 20% CD5/CD19: not done	Aspirate: 27% Trephine: 10% CD5/CD19: 0%
3	Chlorambucil/ prednisolone, cyclophosphamide, fludarabine, DCF	4	Aspirate: 30% Trephine: 25–30% CD5/CD19: 67%	Aspirate: CR Trephine: CR CD5/CD19: 0%
4	Chlorambucil/ epirubicin, fludarabine	6	Aspirate: 20% Trephine: 25–30% CD5/CD19: 14%	Aspirate: CR Trephine: CR CD5/CD19: 0%
5	Chlorambucil/ prednisolone, fludarabine	4	Aspirate: 10% Trephine: 15% CD5/CD19: 54%	Aspirate: CR Trephine: CR CD5/CD19: 0%
6	Chlorambucil/ prednisolone, fludarabine, CHOP	10	Aspirate: 95% Trephine: 30% CD5/CD19: not done	Aspirate: CR Trephine: MRD* CD5/CD19: 2%

*Minimal residual disease detectable as few small foci of infiltration containing 18% CD5/CD19 cells, and PB lymphopenia

Adapted from Dyer *et al*[6].

The Royal Marsden NHS Trust experience within study 005 included assessment of the efficacy of subcutaneous injection in a limited number of patients with fludarabine-resistant or relapsed lymphomas. Four of these heavily pre-treated patients had B-CLL, two had pre-B-cell leukemia (CLL/PL) and one had pro-lymphocytic leukemia (PLL). Campath-1H was administered as an undiluted solution of 10 mg/ml beginning at a unit dose of 10 mg, then rising to 30 mg as three divided doses of no more than 1 ml per injection[7]. All patients were given oral prophylactic cotrimoxazole, and those with a prior history of herpes virus infection received prophylactic acyclovir. The B-PLL patient entered remission, remained in complete response for three months and then underwent transformation to a large cell lymphoma which was fatal.

Durable responses were seen in four patients (median 11 months post-therapy). All seven patients developed a local injection site reaction after the first dose, but subsequent injections were better tolerated. The most significant side-effect was re-activation of cytomegalovirus (CMV) infection seen in three patients; one infection was subclinical and the other two were treated with gancyclovir. Three B-CLL patients achieved partial response, and two were re-treated with a further course of Campath-1H after several months with stable disease and responded a second time. The fourth B-CLL patient showed minimal response and was not suitable for treatment after 6 weeks due to CMV infection. The responses of patients in partial response to a second course of treatment show that it is possible to repeat Campath-1H therapy without additional toxicity.

Fourteen patients were treated with Campath-1H at Long Island Jewish Medical Center as part of study protocol 009[8]. Responses of the whole cohort according to site are shown in Table 4. The durations of response were: 9, 14, 15, 18, 21, 22 and 75 months, and one patient died at 2 months while in partial response.

Table 4. Responses to Campath-1H in heavily treated patients (Study 009)

	Responses to Campath-1H			
	CR		**PR**	
	%	***n***	**%**	***n***
Overall response (*n*=12)	16.6%	2	58%	7
Response by disease site				
Bone marrow (*n*=12)	42%	5	33.3%	4
Spleen (*n*=5)	80%	4	20%	1
Lymph node, small (*n*=6)	100%	6	—	—
Lymph node, bulky (*n*=5)	40%	2	60%	3

* Refers to resolution of lymphocytosis

Three of the responders relapsed more than a year after achieving remission and were re-entered into the study. After re-entry, one patient did not respond to re-treatment, one responded and then relapsed, and the third has been re-treated five times with response and remains on a maintenance dose.

An additional case history reported by Laikon General Hospital, Athens, participating in study 005[9] emphasizes further that Campath-1H re-treatment can continue to provoke a response, in this instance over a 3-year period. While generally, nodal disease is seen to respond less well to Campath-1H than blood or marrow infiltration, in this case, while response in the bone marrow was variable, the regression of lymphadenopathy was consolidated in each of three treatment cycles. The patient was a 55-year-old male who had been treated with chlorambucil with only a minor response, then switched to cyclophosphamide for 8 weeks. Three months later, his disease was progressing with a lymphocyte increase to $169 \times 10^9/l$, a drop in hemoglobin and an increase in lymphadenopathy and splenomegaly. He was then entered into the 005 trial. Treatment was well-tolerated and the response was impressive. Lymphadenopathy was dramatically decreased; a few axillary and inguinal nodes remaining, not greater than 1 cm in diameter as shown in Figure 2. The WBC became normal and the CD19/CD5-positive malignant clone was not detectable in the blood by flow-cytometry after the last infusion of each 12-week cycle. By NCI criteria, complete response was achieved after each cycle of therapy.

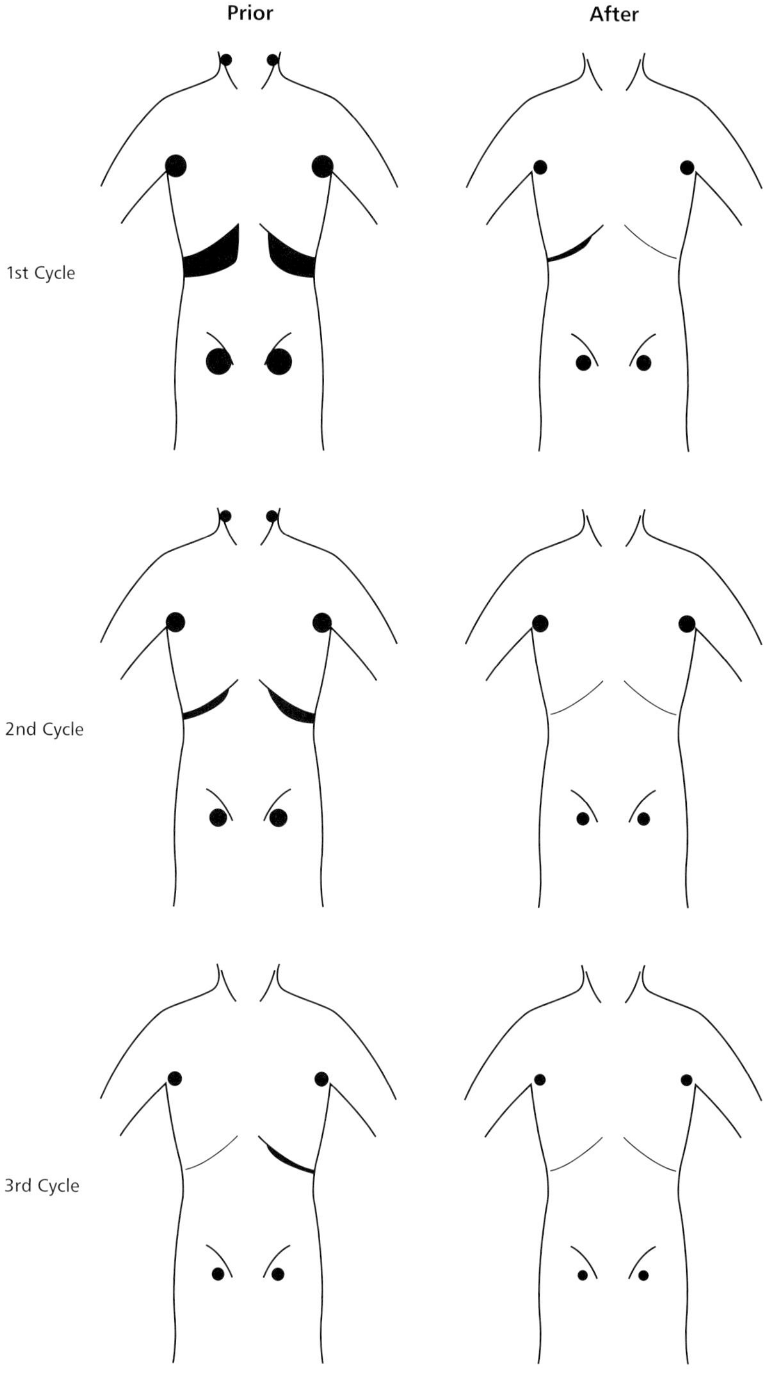

Figure 2. Regression of palpable disease: response of clinically palpable disease prior and after each twelve-week cycle of Campath-1H therapy

The infiltration of the bone marrow by lymphocytes was significantly decreased after each cycle, to approximately 1% after the first cycle, to 20% after the second and to 10% after the third. However, while residual disease was not detectable at the cellular level, PCR of DNA extracted from mononuclear cells detected clone-specific IgG sequence, showing minimal residual disease (MRD) at the molecular level.

This patient remained in clinical complete response for one year after the first cycle of Campath-1H. However, during this time bone marrow infiltration by lymphocytes increased, and when it reached 80%, a second 12-week cycle of Campath-1H treatment was initiated. The results were similar, with a decrease of palpable disease and reduction of WBC count, but residual disease remained in the marrow with an infiltration of 20% shown morphologically and immunophenotypically. Ten months after the end of the second cycle, and because of a slow increase in tumor load, the patient received a third 12-week cycle of Campath-1H. Disease was again controlled, with bone marrow infiltration reduced to approximately 10%. The unavailability of the antibody prevented a possible fourth treatment with Campath-1H. This case history underlines the importance of treating nodal disease before it becomes too bulky.

As with other patients who were re-treated a year or more after first Campath-1H therapy in studies 005 and 009, this case history also demonstrates that toxicity does not increase with subsequent cycles. The side-effects observed during the Athens re-treatment experience were fewer and milder during the second and third cycles of treatment. In addition, during the second and third cycles of treatment, no myelotoxicity or opportunistic infections were observed. The ability to repeat treatments of Campath-1H is a factor which should encourage its investigation in clinical trials as a possible agent of frontline defence in B-CLL.

Within study 005, Campath-1H therapy was used on a small number of previously untreated patients with progressing disease[10]. Nine patients were treated, five receiving the escalating infusions, the remainder having their dosage administered as deep subcutaneous injections, as previously described. Overall, of nine patients, three achieved a CR, five a PR and one developed progressive disease, an overall response rate of 89%.

The results, stratified according to mode of administration are shown in Tables 5 and 6. Administration of Campath-1H by subcutaneous (s.c.) injection has, to date been carried out in very limited numbers of patients, and levels of response seem somewhat lower than with intravenous (i.v.) infusion. It remains available as an option for patients who are unable to continue with infusions due to loss of venous access. Further investigation to directly compare s.c. versus i.v. protocols using randomized trials are required to thoroughly assess the relative merits of these administration methods.

Table 5. Responses to Campath-1H in previously untreated patients[10]
Subcutaneous administration (NCI guidelines)

	CR		PR		SD		PD	
	%	*n*	%	*n*	%	*n*	%	*n*
Overall response (*n*=4)	25%	1	75%	3	—	—	—	—
Response by disease site								
Blood (*n*=4)*	100%	4	—	—	—	—	—	—
Bone marrow (*n*=4)	100%	4	—	—	—	—	—	—
Spleen (*n*=2)	100%	2	—	—	—	—	—	—
Lymph node (*n*=4)	25%	1	75%	3	—	—	—	—

*Refers to resolution of lymphocytosis

Table 6. Responses to Campath-1H in previously untreated patients[10]
Intravenous administration (NCI guidelines)

	CR		PR		SD		PD	
	%	*n*	%	*n*	%	*n*	%	*n*
Overall response (*n*=5)	40%	2	40%	2	—	—	20%	1
Response by disease site								
Blood (*n*=5)*	100%	5	—	—	—	—	—	—
Bone marrow (*n*=5)	60%	3	20%	1	20%	1	—	—
Spleen (*n*=4)	50%	2	50%	2	—	—	—	—
Lymph node (*n*=4)	50%	2	25%	1	—	—	25%	1

*Refers to resolution of lymphocytosis

Hematological toxicity was mild in all these patients; grade 3 neutropenia occurred in one patient, grade 2 in two patients and grade 1 in a single patient, while the remainder showed no reduction of granulocytes. Only one patient experienced a transient grade 1 thrombocytopenia, with platelet levels remaining stable or increasing during treatment in all other patients.

Few infections were seen in this group of patients. One patient developed a CMV pneumonitis, but no other serious side-effects were seen. The authors suggest that this was likely to be due to the good general condition of this cohort compared with heavily pre-treated patients with prolonged underlying disease. Campath-1H has further advantages as an agent of first-line defence since it does not exert its effects within the cell, is not subject to variations in metabolism of the malignant cells and unlike alkylating agents or purine analogues, is not potentially mutagenic. Full assessment of Campath-1H as frontline therapy will rely upon trials assessing its value in large numbers of patients.

As yet, the largest cohort treated with Campath-1H to date is of heavily pre-treated patients all of whom had relapsed or refractory disease after multiple treatments and had all failed to respond or relapsed subsequent to fludarabine treatment. Currently, fludarabine is the agent of last defence. The prognosis for such patients is poor, with median survival estimated to be nine months[11]. Study 211 enrolled 93 such patients in a multi-center trial across Europe and the USA[12]. In order to be eligible for this trial, patients had to have been treated with an alkylating agent, and to have documented failure of treatment with fludarabine-containing regimens. The median number of prior treatments was three (range, 2–7). A diagnosis of B-CLL (CD5+ and CD19+) in progression was required for inclusion, as shown.

Campath-1H Study 211. B-CLL inclusion criteria

- Rai stage III or IV
- Rai stage 0–II with at least **one** of
  - Anemia
  - Thrombocytopenia
  - Autoimmune anemia

continued on page 82

- Autoimmune thrombocytopenia
- Massive or progressive splenomegaly
- Progressive lymphocytosis
  - Increase > 50% in two months
  - Lymphocyte count > 100,000 mm^3
  - B-symptoms

Campath-1H Study 211. Patient demographics

- 76% of enrolled patients had advanced disease (Rai stages III to IV)
- 30% had B-symptoms (night sweats; fatigue; malaise; fever)
- 79% of patients were male
- 56 patients received the full 12 week course as planned
- Median age 66 (range 32 to 86 years)
- Median number of prior treatments 3 (range 2–7)

The most common adverse events in these patients were fever and rigors (89%), nausea and vomiting (50%), rash (33%), fatigue (29%) and dyspnea (24%) with the vast majority of these being grade 1 or 2 severity. Neutropenias and thrombocytopenias occurred in half the enrolled patients, usually improving within the first 1–2 months of discontinuing therapy. Infection occurred in 56% of patients with one third of these being grade 3–5, as shown. Most infections occurred in the first 2 months and rapidly diminished after therapy was completed.

Campath-1H Study 211. Incidence of grade 3–5 infections

- Pneumonia (5%)
- CMV (2%)
- *Candida* (2%)
- Septicemia (2%)
- Others (4%)

The overall intent-to-treat response rate was 33% (95% CI: 24–43%) with 2 (2%) complete responses, 29 (31%) partial responses and 55 (59%) stable disease. These latter patients with stable disease according to NCI criteria did show anti-tumor responses in the peripheral blood (97%), lymph nodes (62%), liver (73%) and spleen (71%). Similarly, the report of data of 10 patients enrolled at a single center within study 211, shown in Table 7, show that bone marrow and spleen are particularly responsive sites. Of the seven responders in this patient group, one relapsed at six months, while the remaining six were still in remission at 10 (1 patient), 11 (3 patients) and 12 months (2 patients)[8], exceeding the predicted life expectancy of heavily pre-treated patients (median 9 months)[11].

Table 7. Responses to Campath-1H in heavily treated patients[8] (NCI guidelines) study 211, Long Island Jewish Medical Center

	CR		PR	
	%	*n*	%	*n*
Overall response (*n*=10)	20%	2	50%	5
Response by disease site				
Bone marrow (*n*=10)	50%	5	20%	2
Spleen (*n*=7)	86%	6	14.2%	1
Lymph node, small (*n*=6)	—	—	83.3%	5

* Refers to resolution of lymphocytosis

The ability to clear peripheral blood, and/or marrow is of particular significance since it may allow certain patients to proceed to bone marrow transplantation.

A preliminary report from Leeds University and Nottingham City Hospital, participating in studies 005 and 211 within the UK, shows that of the 29 B-CLL patients who have received the escalating dosage of Campath-1H in these centers, seven have now gone on to bone marrow transplantation[13], discussed further in Chapter 5. Campath-1H did not interfere with peripheral blood stem cell mobilization and harvesting and has greatly increased the feasibility of bone marrow transplantation for B-CLL patients.

Response to therapy in these 29 patients was analyzed by four-color flow cytometry in addition to conventional assessment. Seventeen (59%) patients responded to therapy, with ten (34%) achieving a complete remission by NCI criteria. Of these ten, five had malignant cells detectable by flow cytometry, while five had no detectable cells either by flow cytometry or by PCR amplification of IgG heavy chain rearrangement specific for the malignant clone. As with other cohorts, significant lymphadenopathy predicted a worse response, since 14 out of 17 patients without nodal disease responded compared with three out of 12 patients with bulky nodal disease.

Campath-1H in refractory B-CLL: summary

- Highly active
- Relatively safe
- Re-treatment possible
- Most effective before nodal disease becomes bulky

Conclusions

Overall, these studies demonstrate that Campath-1H is highly active in patients with B-CLL in progression after multiple treatments including fludarabine. They demonstrate that it is possible to re-treat with Campath-1H without any increase in toxicity and that such re-treatment can evoke further responses. They further show that therapy is best initiated before the development of bulky disease. Campath-1H did not interfere with peripheral blood stem cell mobilization and harvesting and has greatly increased the feasibility of bone marrow transplantation for B-CLL patients and brought the goal of 'true' molecular remission for such patients within reach.

Reference List

1. Johnson S, Smith AG, Loffler H, Osby E, Juliusson G, Emmerich B, Wyld PJ, Hiddemann W. Multicentre prospective randomised trial of fludarabine versus cyclophosphamide, doxorubicin, and prednisone (CAP) for treatment of advanced-stage chronic lymphocytic leukaemia. The French Cooperative Group on CLL *Lancet.* 1996;347:1432–1438

2. Foran JM, Rohatiner AZ, Coiffier B, Barbui T, Johnson SA, Hiddemann W, Radford JA, Norton AJ, Tollerfield SM, Wilson MP, Lister TA. Multicenter phase II study of fludarabine phosphate for patients with newly diagnosed lymphoplasmacytoid lymphoma, Waldenström's macroglobulinemia, and mantle-cell lymphoma. *J Clin Oncol.* 1999;17:546–553

3. Hansen MM, Andersen E, Christensen BE, Christiansen I, Geisler C, Kristensen D, Jensen KB, Junker P. CHOP versus prednisolone + chlorambucil in chronic lymphocytic leukemia (CLL): preliminary results of a randomized multicenter study. *Nouv Rev Fr Hematol.* 1988;30:433–436

4. Osterborg A, Dyer MJ, Bunjes D, Pangalis GA, Bastion Y, Catovsky D, Mellstedt H. Phase II multicenter study of human CD52 antibody in previously treated chronic lymphocytic leukemia. European Study Group of CAMPATH-1H Treatment in Chronic Lymphocytic Leukemia. *J Clin Oncol.* 1997;15:1567–1574

5. Rawstron AC, Davies FE, Evans P, Morgan GJ, Jamil A, Galvin MC, Haynes AP, Hale G, Hillmen P. Campath1H therapy for patients with refractory chronic lymphocytic leukemia (CLL). *Blood.* 1997;90(Suppl 1): (abstract 2356)

6. Dyer MJ, Kelsey SM, Mackay HJ, Emmett E, Thornton P, Hale G, Waldmann H, Newland AC, Catovsky D. *In vivo* 'purging' of residual disease in CLL with Campath-1H. *Br J Haematol.* 1997;97:669–672

7. Bowen AL, Zomas A, Emmett E, Matutes E, Dyer MJ, Catovsky D. Subcutaneous CAMPATH-1H in fludarabine-resistant/relapsed chronic lymphocytic and B-prolymphocytic leukaemia. *Br J Haematol.* 1997;96:617–619

8. Hoffman M, Janson D, Rai K. Analysis of response to Campath-1H in patients with B-CLL progressing after fludarabine therapy. *Hematol Cell Ther* (IWCLL 1999). 2000;42:109 (abstract P129)

9. Pangalis GA, Dimopoulou MN, Angelopoulou MK, Siakantaris MP. Campath-1H in B-chronic lymphocytic leukemia: report on a patient treated thrice in a 3 year period. *Med Oncol.* 2000;17:70–73

10. Osterborg A, Fassas AS, Anagnostopoulos A, Dyer MJ, Catovsky D, Mellstedt H. Humanized CD52 monoclonal antibody Campath-1H as first-line treatment in chronic lymphocytic leukaemia. *Br J Haematol.* 1996;93:151–153

11. Keating M, O'Brien S, Plunkett W, Koller C, Beran M, Lerner S, Kantarjian H. Results of first salvage therapy for patients refractory to a Fludara regimen in chronic lymphocytic leukemia. *Leuk Lymphoma.* (In press)

12. Keating MJ, Byrd J, Rai K, Flinn I, Jain V, Binet JL, Bolin R, Hillmen P, Hutchinson M. Campath-1H Collaborative Study Group. Multicenter study of Campath-1H in patients with chronic lymphocytic leukemia (B-CLL) refractory to fludarabine. *Blood.* 1999;94: (abstract 3118)

13. Kennedy SM, Rawstron AC, Evans P, English A, Haynes AP, Russell NH, Byrne B, Hale G, Morgan GJ, Hillmen P. Campath-IH therapy in 29 patients with refractory CLL: 'true' complete remission is an attainable goal. *Blood.* 1999;94:603a (abstract 2683)

5

The Role of Campath-1H Prior to BMT in Refractory B-CLL

The use of Campath-1H in patients with B-CLL can be regarded, not only as a treatment in its own right, reducing tumor cells, but also as a preparative regimen for bone marrow transplantation (BMT) with potential for effecting a cure.

The long natural history of B-CLL, the fact that most sufferers are elderly and the procedure-related mortality have been considerable deterrents to the use of BMT in this disease. Some procedure-related problems occur when conventional stem cell transplantation is preceded by high-dose conditioning and/or total body irradiation designed to control the malignancy, associated with a high incidence of acute and long-term side-effects. These factors have largely prevented the use of BMT, particularly allografting with its risk of GVHD, for patients older than 55 years. High-dose regimens are now being increasingly replaced by procedures which are minimally immunosuppressive rather than totally myeloablative and which are usually based on fludarabine, often in combination with cyclophosphamide[1-3]. Conveniently, there is substantial overlap between these new preparative regimens and the drug schedules most effective in reducing tumor burden in B-CLL. In one sense, Campath-1H can itself be regarded as a form of non-myeloablative immunosuppressive BMT conditioning.

The introduction of an escalating dose regimen using Campath-1H to purge malignant cells *in vivo* also coincides with a number of other improvements in transplant procedures and in post-transplant supportive care, and the achievement of a deeper understanding of the nature of engraftment and the reconstitution of the immune system it entails.

The principles behind BMT

BMT can be viewed as a natural form of gene therapy to replace a defective cell or enzyme with a functional and normally regulated one, not only in malignancies but in inherited disease. Experience gained in some of the wider applications of BMT is now contributing to an understanding of processes involved in the promotion and speed of engraftment, the nature of GVHD, and the importance of the graft-versus-leukemia (GVL) effect.

Engraftment

The speed of engraftment depends on the concentration of hematopoietic progenitor cells in the transplant. Such cells can be derived from bone marrow, or may be obtained from peripheral blood[4,5], following mobilization using G-CSF[6]. The data accumulating, showing that peripheral blood can be effective as a source of stem cells[7–10], have particular potential for B-CLL autografting, since in many B-CLL patients, malignant cells can be more readily cleared in the blood than in the marrow[4,11].

There may be an optimum dosage of stem cells (usually assessed using CD34 as a marker), since doses of less than 4×10^6/kg are associated with a poor prognosis[8,12]. Doses greater than 7×10^6/kg may facilitate allogeneic engraftment by tolerization, an effect which may be due to the failure of CD34 cells to present costimulatory molecules[13,14]. However, in the case of autologous transplantation megadosing brings with it an increased risk of reintroduction of malignant cells[15]. Allogeneic transplants, on the other hand, overcome the problem of possible malignant contamination. Allografts may also be necessary instead of autografts in CLL if the extent of the disease or the nature of prior treatment makes it difficult to harvest sufficient quantities of the patient's own stem cells. Allogeneic transplantation is both riskier, because of GVHD, and has benefits, in that the donor cells may recognize any residual leukemic cells as foreign and so mount an immune attack to eradicate them; the GVL effect. The exact nature of the GVL effect, as discussed below, is not yet clear, but many attempts are being made to harness its potential in leukemia/lymphoma, including in B-CLL.

Graft-versus-host disease

This is a distressing and potentially fatal condition occurring after allogeneic transplantation in which T-cells contributed by the donor mount a pervasive inflammatory attack on host tissues, and occurs in two distinct forms: acute and chronic.

Most data on GVHD derive from allografts between HLA-matched siblings. Acute GVHD usually begins within 2 weeks following a transplant, and may last for 3 months, affecting the skin, liver, stomach, and/or intestines. The earliest signs of acute GVHD are a skin rash that appears on the hand, feet and face. The rash may spread to other parts of the body and in severe cases develop into a general blistering red rash. Severe forms of acute GVHD of the stomach and/or intestines result in patients developing large amounts of watery or bloody diarrhea with cramping. Jaundice indicates that GVHD involves the liver. Acute GVHD may be life-threatening, but the milder cases respond to treatment with steroids.

Acute GVHD

- Rashes
- Blisters
- Fever
- Diarrhea/cramping
- Jaundice
- In severe cases, toxic shock

Chronic GVHD is seen in approximately 40% of patients after allogeneic transplant, usually beginning 2–3 months post-transplant. Its precise causes are unclear but are related to the balance of T-cell subsets from host and recipient as the new chimeric immune system is reconstituted. It resembles many spontaneously occurring auto-immune disorders. Most patients experience skin and mouth symptoms and because chronic GVHD is capable of attacking almost any body organ there can be a wide variety of additional symptoms.

The most serious threat to health comes from the reduced ability to fight infection which is associated with chronic GVHD. However, the deeply unpleasant nature of the other symptoms makes the non-life-threatening aspects of the disease extremely hard for patients to bear and puts pressure on the physician to use BMT regimens with a reduced risk of developing chronic GVHD.

Chronic GVHD

- Pebbly raised rash 'alligator skin'
- Skin discoloration, increased and/or decreased pigmentation
- Alopecia and/or premature greying
- Decreased ability to sweat
- Dry mouth, food sensitivity
- Dry/reddened eyes
- Jaundice
- Malaise
- Fatigue
- GVHD can attack almost any body organ: wide variability in additional symptoms

Graft-versus-leukemia effects

Many studies have demonstrated that patients who survive have a decreased risk of relapse compared to patients receiving autografts, or grafts from identical twins, or those who simply fail to develop any form of GVHD. These data imply that host T-cells can attack leukemia cells and first indicated the existence of graft-versus-leukemia effects. Their exact nature is unclear.

A key question which remains to be answered is whether the same donor T-cell subsets are responsible for GVHD and GVL. If so, then the best case scenario for a patient may be to experience controlled GVHD as the price of protection from leukemic relapse. However, if different T-cell subsets mount immune responses against tumor and against host tissue, there remains the possibility that the GVL effect can be evoked without the occurrence of GVHD. CD4[16] and CD3[17] cells have been implicated in the GVL effect and CD6[18], CD8[19,20] and NK cells[21] in engraftment and GVHD, and their precise roles are under investigation.

In an ideal situation it would be possible to harness GVL effects without promoting GVHD, or slowing engraftment. Research, much of it using murine models, is being carried out to determine which T-cells are responsible for these functions and whether GVL without GVHD is feasible.

Engraftment is highly dependent upon the balance between donor and host T-cell subsets. Rejection occurs if host T-cells predominate. One model holds CD8 cells responsible, shown to prevent marrow graft rejection in mice primarily by generating cytotoxic T-lymphocytes. Dividing CD8 cells into subsets which express αβ or γδ T-cell receptors (TCR+) and those which do not (TCR-) has revealed that both subsets can facilitate engraftment in mice[22] and have different effects on GVHD. The TCR+ cells subset eliminated recipient T-cells and the TCR- subset, which may be lymphoid dendritic cells, did not. TCR-/CD8+ cells could overcome the engraftment barrier created by recipient NK cells and were most effective when limited numbers of highly enriched progenitor cells were used. Additional studies in mice have used highly selected hematopoietic stem cells in attempts to identify populations that facilitate engraftment[23,24]. However, a pivotal role for CD8+ subsets has yet to be substantiated in humans, and may prove to be system-specific.

Since graft-versus-leukemia effects may be based in a direct attack against tumor-specific antigens they may therefore require such antigens to be highly expressed. Alternatively donor effects in leukemia may be a more general reaction in which tumor cells expressing low-level markers are recognized in the presence of co-stimulatory molecules, stimuli to which the host immune system has become tolerant. GVL effects can be most clearly seen in CML[25] in which donor lymphocyte infusions (DLI) can reliably induce disease remission, and appear to be augmented with increased HLA disparity between donor and recipient[26]. Unlike Ph+ve CML cells which express the tumor-specific marker BCR-ABL, CLL cells do not all possess the same target antigen. The antigenic target for the T-cell response in CML has not been conclusively demonstrated to be BCR-ABL, however, and patients in remission after DLI develop

B-cell-mediated immunity, targeting a range of CML-associated products not solely BCR-ABL[27].

Preliminary evidence indicates that a GVL effect does exist in CLL[28-30], as shown by DLI induced remissions in small numbers of patients.

While some data seem to offer the hope that it may be possible to identify cells capable of eliciting GVL in the absence of GVHD[31] and work on dissecting out roles of T-cell subpopulations is continuing, the two effects may prove to be inextricably linked, and the answer to the problem of GVHD may be to control it, eliminating the life-threatening and debilitating forms, while harnessing any beneficial effects of mild forms.

The Campath series of antibodies have a substantial history of use in BMT because of their ability to control GVHD in this way and so avoid a major cause of treatment-related morbidity and mortality in allografting.

T-cell depletion

Removal of T-cells

Selection	Purging

• Immunoselection
  • Magnetic beads
  • Avidin-biotin immunoaffinity column
	• Anti-CD52 (Campath)
	  • Monoclonal cocktail; Anti-CD2, CD3, CD8
	  • Elutriation
	  • E-rosetting

GVHD can be minimized or avoided by depleting donor cells of T-cells, and many ways have been developed to achieve this. Such methods each have their own advantages and disadvantages. Any depletion method which reduces stem cell load may be unadvisable if limited sources of stem cells are available, since this may delay engraftment or increase the risk of graft failure. Widely used methods remove CD52-bearing T- and B-cells using Campath antibodies, which have the advantage that 100% stem cells are retained.

T-cell depletion methods fall into two groups; indirect depletion of T-cells by selection of CD34+ stem cells, and direct purging of T-cells. Methods to carry out the latter are very varied. They include physical separation of monocytes from B- and T-cells using centrifugal counterflow elutriation[32], or using E-rosetting to remove T-cells[10,33]. While most of the other methods remove 98–99% T-cells, elutriation may remove as little as 80% so retaining a risk of GVHD[34,35]. It also has the disadvantage that it reduces CD34+ cell counts considerably[36] with up to 75% of the CD34+ cells being lost in the small lymphocyte fraction[37].

E-rosetting, in which bone marrow is exposed to sequential soyabean lectin followed by agglutination in the presence of sheep red blood cells, is effective but is relatively complex to administer, and is not widely available.

Other more specific methods purge by binding cells carrying lymphocyte-specific cell markers using cocktails composed of multiple antibodies[24,33,38], although at present there is no combination which has managed to achieve the ideal of GVL and rapid engraftment without GVHD.

Of these methods Campath antibodies are both simple and extremely effective options to reduce GVHD. The monoclonals can be used to condition the recipient using an intravenous infusion of Campath-1G ‘in the bag’ with no further manipulation, with or without depleting the graft using Campath-1M plus complement[39]. Depletion of donor T-cells alone gives excellent protection against GVHD but can increase the incidence of graft failure due to rejection by the host. Graft rejection can be partly overcome by using Campath-1G *in vivo*[39–42]. Alternatively, a single dose of Campath-1G or 1H added to donor marrow can accomplish both conditioning and graft depletion, since excess antibody is infused along with the graft, giving sufficient depletion by opsonization *in vivo* to prevent rejection in many patients[43]. Serum levels of Campath may also be supplemented after transplant to increase levels of purging *in vivo*[44].

In a comparison of Campath-1M/complement with direct CD34+ selection Clarke *et al.* found that such graft depletion produced very similar CD34+ recovery and that the proliferative potential of the Campath-derived cells as measured using colonies produced after cytokine stimulus were greater, shown in Table 1[45]. The residual fraction after CD34+ immunoselection contains such T-cell subsets as CD3 or CD8, and can be retained and further fractionated for possible use as a donor lymphocyte infusion (DLI) to rescue in the event of relapse.

Loss of cells is the main disadvantage of CD34+ selection with recoveries ranging from 45% to 75%[46].

Table 1. Stem cell recovery

	Campath-1M	CD34+ Immunoselection
CD34+ recovery	50% (± 7%)	55% (± 12%)
CFU-GM 7	8% (± 20%)	44% (± 12%)
BFU-E	79% (± 18%)	42% (± 13%)
T-cell-depletion	98.4 (± 1.9%)	99.8% (±0.2%)

Use of Campath antibodies *ex vivo* retains 100% CD34+ cells, and these high recoveries allow 20–30% of the graft to be set aside for DLI. A further advantage over direct selection is that progenitor cells which are CD34– are not depleted.

This is of current interest because attention has recently been directed at the phenotype of progenitor cell populations, since it appears that stem cells exist which possess full reconstitutive capacity and yet do not express CD34 on their surface[46].

The first evidence that selecting CD34+ cells for transplant might be excluding another population of stem cells was obtained in mice, where a CD34– cell was detected which had full engrafting capacity[47]. A human equivalent to these cells was then found[48], and these primitive cells were also been correlated with a primitive population of cells found in mouse, monkey and man which exclude drugs and toxins due to high expression of the multi-drug-resistance (MDR) trans-membrane pumps[49]. The biology of CD34 positive and negative cells was further elucidated by the demonstration that CD34 expression is reversible in stem cells, that CD34– cells can be induced to express CD34 and that, in the mouse, CD34+ cells can revert to a CD34– phenotype after transplantation and retain secondary, multilineage engraftment capacity[50]. When freshly isolated, these CD34– cells have low engraftment capacity, but when expanded *in vitro* rapidly induce CD34 expression and multilineage potential[51]. The most provocative finding with regard to the question of whether to select directly or indirectly for CD34+ cells is the suggestion that the CD34– stem cells are not so easily exhausted as CD34+ cells in a pre-immune fetal transplantation model[52,53]. This work suggests that human CD34– cells act as a reservoir for production of CD34+ cells and may have longer or more durable reconstitution capabilities. This means that they may be significant, post-transplant, in the long-term replenishment of normal hematopoiesis. Until the nature, and the quantitative benefits, of this alternative source of stem cells have been fully established, it may be prudent to use selection methods that deplete mature lymphocytes rather than those which select for CD34+ alone.

In addition to the risk of GVHD, transplantation carries a further risk; that of Epstein–Barr virus-triggered (EBV) lymphoproliferative disease, which may be fatal.

In autologous transplantation, this is relatively rare and occurs by opportunistic establishment of endogenous virus during the period of severe immunodepletion. In these cases, a rapid engraftment, promoted by an optimum stem cell load in the graft, will lower this risk.

In allogeneic transplantation, there is the further risk that EBV may be introduced with the donor B-lymphocytes. Extensive surveys reviewing nearly 20,000 transplants have shown that increased risk of this secondary malignancy is associated with T-cell depletion compared with the infusion of unmanipulated marrow[54,55]. Dissecting out the risks associated with different methods of T-cell depletion shows that the risk is highest when strategies are used which retain B-cell populations, as is the case in E-rosetting or using antibodies directed against markers specific to T-cells, and lowest when methods are used which also eliminate introduction of donor B-cells, such as the Campath series of antibodies, elutriation, or direct selection of stem cells. In a comparison of E-rosetting versus Campath in 2582 patients, the risk was as high as 29% in the E-rosette group and reduced to 1.3% in the Campath group, which is little different from the rate in patients transplanted with unmodified marrow[56]. The additional depletion of B-cells appears to be beneficial, possibly because it reduces virus load, or because it reduces virus target until the time when T-cells begin to regenerate.

Campath depletion of T-cells

Summary

✓ Low risk of EBV-triggered secondary malignancy
✓ No loss of CD34 negative stem cells
✓ Good stem cell recovery
✓ Does not interfere with PBSC mobilization
✓ Reduces GVDH
× Does not allow separate collection of T-subsets for DLI
× May increase risk of relapse

While Campath-1G and 1H can consistently control GVHD and promote engraftment across a range of leukemias and lymphomas, the disadvantages which remain are those of leukemic relapse, most prominent after T-cell depletion in CML[57], and susceptibility to infection during immune reconstitution. Patients who receive T-cell-depleted bone marrow transplants are at risk from infections during the first year post-transplant (Geoff Hale and CAMPATH users, unpublished work). A study of immune reconstitution after T-cell-depleted PBSC transplantation showed that while total T-cell counts reached the normal range, CD4+ counts remained subnormal 1 year post-transplant[58]. Immune recovery is an area which requires to be studied in detail in more patient over a longer term.

BMT in B-CLL to date

As shown in Tables 2 and 4, (updated from Flynn & Vogelsang, 1998)[59], when CLL patients are offered BMT at a relatively young age, both autologous and allogeneic transplants can achieve success in promoting engraftment and remission.

Table 2. Autologous bone marrow transplant for CLL

Patients (*n*)	Age	Prior therapies (*n*)	Remission	Event-free survival (months)	Overall survival (median follow up in months)	Ref
12	45 (27–54)	3 (1–4)	10/11 CR 1NE	10/12, 83% (6, 2-31)	11/12, 92% (6, 2–31)	60
11	59 (37–66)	3 (2–5)	6/11 CR, 55% 4/11 nCR, 36% 1/11 PR	3/11, 27% (4–29)	6/11, 55% (10)	61

CR, Complete remission; PR, Partial remission; nCR, Nodular complete remission

The study carried out by Rabinowe *et al.* (reference 60, Table 2) used a preparative regimen consisting of high-dose cyclophosphamide and total body irradiation (TBI) and grafted 20 patients, eight of whom received autografts, re-infused after purging with multiple monoclonal antibodies, and 12 of whom received T-cell-depleted allografts from HLA- matched siblings. Remissions were assessed at hematological level and at the molecular level using detection of clonal IgG rearrangements. In the autologous group, ten patients achieved CR, and in the allogeneic group seven achieved CR with the eighth showing a hematological remission with <10% marrow involvement. Similarly, of 11 patients receiving autografts after purging using an anti-CD19 monoclonal antibody[61], six patients achieved CR. Post-transplant mortality in these patients remained high, however, since out of these six patients, two patients died in CR, one transformed to Richter's syndrome eight months after transplant and one patient relapsed twelve months after transplant.

Additional studies of autologous transplantation in B-CLL, using standard high-dose preparative regimens on young patient cohorts (median age 49 years, range 29–61)[62] have confirmed the rapid engraftment possible with peripheral blood stem cells (PBSC) (13 patients) compared with bone marrow (three patients). Remission was confirmed at the molecular level using PCR to detect clone-specific IgG rearrangements. Single case studies have also successfully performed autologous transplantation in B-CLL after high dose chlorambucil in a 49-year-old patient with auto-immune complications[63]. Similarly, mobilized PBSC were observed to engraft rapidly[64] whether or not T-cell depletion by CD34+ selection was carried out.

One of the problems with autologous transplantation using PBSC in patients with advanced B-CLL is that even with the increased numbers of stem cells it is possible to harvest using cytokine mobilization, it may not be possible to obtain sufficient stem cells for manipulation and rapid engraftment. In three of 17 patients studied by Scime *et al.*[65], harvest was insufficient. They noted that stem cell yield was greater in patients who had achieved a complete response prior to transplant than in those in PR.

The increasing use of non-myeloablative conditioning regimens may open the way for more reliable harvests and for older patients to be successfully given autografts.

Typical non-myeloablative regimen

Autografts

In vivo conditioning:

- Cyclophosphamide 60 mg/kg (days –7 and –6)
- Fludarabine 25 mg/m^2 (days –5 to –1)
- Cyclosporine was started on day –4 as host-versus-graft (HVG) prophylaxis

However, while these new regimens are proving valuable as conditioning for allografts[29], the use of purine analogues may compromise the yield of stem cells from some patients, as demonstrated by Schey *et al.*[66], a study in which ten B-CLL patients were treated. Two of the ten did not mobilize sufficient stem cells to allow selection to be carried out. Of the eight in whom selection of harvested cells was undertaken, only five had an adequate yield post-selection to allow them to proceed to transplantation and so underwent transplantation with a mix of selected and unselected 'backup' cells.

In contrast, Campath-1H did not interfere with peripheral blood stem cell mobilization or harvesting in studies at the Royal Marsden NHS Trust, as discussed in Chapter 4. Purity of peripheral blood stem cells was demonstrated to be sufficient for subsequent autologous transplantation in five of six patients[67], and all six gave good yields. This group had been treated to maximum response with purine analogues (either fludarabine or pentostatin) but had retained persistent leukemic infiltration of both blood and bone marrow. Campath-1H treatment allowed five patients to achieve complete hematological remission with no detectable CD5+/CD19+ cells, of whom two went on to successful autologous transplantation. Stem cell harvest data are shown in Table 3 (patient numbers correlate to those in Table 3, Chapter 4).

Table 3. Peripheral blood stem cell harvests after Campath-1H treatment: Royal Marsden experience

Patients (*n*)	BM infiltration after Campath-1H	Yield of cells PBSC harvest(/kg)	%CD5/CD19 in PBSC harvest	Outcome after Campath-1H (duration)
1	Aspirate: CR Trephine: CR CD5+/CD19+: 1%	MNCS: 2.25 $\times 10^8$ CD34+:3.43 $\times 10^6$	55%	GPR 12 months post transplant: CD5+/CD19+30% BM
2	Aspirate: 27% Trephine: 10% CD5+/CD19+: 0%	MNCS: 2.32 $\times 10^8$ CD34+: 4.43 $\times 10^6$	33%	CR 10 months post transplant CD5+/CD19+38% in PB with normal count at 5 months
3	Aspirate: CR Trephine:CR CD5+/CD19+: 0%	MNCS: 1.18 $\times 10^8$ CD34+: 0.86 $\times 10^6$	0%	CR for 7 months: CD5+/CD19+ 40% at 5 months; BM/PB relapse at 7 months
4	Aspirate: CR Trephine: CR CD5+/CD19+ 0%:	MNCS: 3.6 $\times 10^8$ CD34+:1.14 $\times 10^6$	4%	CR 12 months
5	Aspirate: CR Trephine: CR CD5+/CD19+: 0%	MNCS: 3.5 $\times 10^8$ CD34+: 1.49 $\times 10^6$	0%	CR: 9 months +
6	Aspirate: CR Trephine: MRD* CD5+/CD19+: 2%	MNCS: 3.4 $\times 10^8$ CD34+: 0.2 $\times 10^6$	Not tested	GPR: matched unrelated BMT 5 months later; Alive 9 months+

MNCS, mononuclear cells; BM, bone marrow; PBSC, peripheral blood stem cells; GPR, good partial response. *MRD, minimal residual disease (few small foci of infiltration) and peripheral blood lymphopenia with 48% CD5+/CD19+ cells

Adapted from Dyer *et al*[67].

Two patients with a previously rapid clinical course went immediately on to high-dose BEAM therapy (BCNU, etoposide, Ara-C and melphalan) followed by autologous transplantation with successful rapid engraftment. In patients 3–5, with no or minimal contamination from malignant cells, it was elected to observe subsequent progress before transplantation. The sixth patient who retained minimal residual disease went on to allogeneic transplantation from a matched unrelated donor after 5 months.

The finding that Campath-1H does not interfere with mobilization or stem cell harvesting has been confirmed by a recent report of seven patients who proceeded to autologous PBSCT after Campath-1H therapy[68]. Of the seven, six were alive at a median of 10 months post-transplant (range 4–24). Two of these patients improved to have no detectable disease by four-color flow cytometry, capable of detecting 1 in 10,000 cells, on repeated analysis (21, 23 and 34 months post-Campath-1H treatment).

Autologous transplantation

107 patients reviewed

- TBI in 63%
- Purging in 59%
- PBSCT in 78%
- CR achieved in 90%
- Estimated survival at 2 years 84%
- 21 patients relapsed median 23 months (range 7–48)

A review of 107 patients from 15 centers[69] has recently assessed the long-term benefits of autologous transplantation in B-CLL, using protocols which did not include Campath antibodies, as shown, and concluded that while overall survival is improved over conventional treatment, this may be due to unavoidable selection bias. The authors further concluded that the continuous pattern of relapses suggests that autologous BMT does not cure B-CLL. Current practise in which residual disease is analyzed at the cellular or molecular level may identify a subset of patients who have achieved true remission. However, for patients who have residual disease at transplant, autologous grafting may not be the best option.

Allogeneic transplantation for B-CLL may decrease relapse due to the potential GVL eradication of residual malignant cells. It also has the advantage that marrow and/or stem cell harvesting of high numbers of donor stem cells is possible. Nevertheless, these advantages are offset by higher treatment-related risks.

Table 4. Allogeneic bone marrow transplant for LGL/CLL

No of patients	Age median (range)	No of prior therapies	Remission	Event-free survival (months)	Overall survival (median follow up in months)	Ref
26	44 (21–49)	NA	19/26 PR (54%)	14/26	11/26 42.3%	70
54	41 (21–58)	NA	38/54 HR (70%)	23/54, 43% (27, 5–80)	24/54, 44% (27, 5–80)	71
11	42 (25–55)	3 (1–4)	7/11 CR (64%)	10/11, 91% (11, 2–36)	10/11, 91% 11, 2–36)	61
8	40 (31–54)	2.5 (1–6)	7/8 CR (88%) 8/8 HR (110%)	7/8, 88% (12, 6–18)	6/8, 75% (12, 6–18)	60
29 (10 CLL)	42 (20–25)	NA	23/29 CR (79%)	13/29, 44% (29, 1–85)	17/29, 58.6% (29, 1–85)	72

CR, Complete remission; PR, Partial remission; HR, Hematological remission

In the earliest of the allograft studies shown in Table 4, in which 26 patients received treatment, while remissions were achieved, the treatment-related mortality was considerable. Twelve patients died of early complications of the transplant (GVHD, infection, hemorrhage, etc) while only three died of immune progression. The largest series of allografts of a cohort of 54 patients[71] had 30 deaths, 25 of which were treatment related and generally due to GVHD.

As shown in the table, advances in the reduction of GVHD are improving these results[61,72]. With regard to survival, the follow-up is too short in most reported cases to say for sure whether the remissions are durable enough to constitute a cure. However, analysis of blood samples at the molecular level[73], which shows that the IgG rearrangement specific to the malignant clone is absent after transplant, is very encouraging.

Progress in T-cell depletion methodology is increasingly allowing patients to be transplanted with unrelated donors[74], and even allowing manipulation of GVHD to provoke remission post transplant[75,76].

The development of non-myeloablative conditioning regimens, represents a considerable advance for allogeneic transplantation[29,77,78]. Such regimens have produced encouraging results in malignant lymphoma[79] with improvements in transplant-related toxicity, in a high-risk patient cohort with heavily pre-treated advanced disease.

While such studies have demonstrated impressive engraftment, GVHD remains a significant problem. The incidence of grade II–IV acute GVHD is 38%–60% and it is the primary cause of death in some patients.

Mini-BEAM-Campath

Allografts (Cull *et al.* 2000[80])

In vivo conditioning:

- Campath-1H 10 mg/day i.v. (days –5 to –1)
- BCNU 300 mg/m^2 (day –6)
- Cytosine arabinoside 200 mg/m^2 (day –5 to –2)
- Melphalan 140 mg/m^2 (day –1)
- Methotrexate was given on days 1, 3 and 6 and cyclosporine was started on day –1 as GVHD prophylaxis

In vitro grafts:

- Sibling PBSC donors had been G-CSF mobilized days –4 to 0,
- PBSC grafts contained a median of 7 million CD34+/kg
- BM grafts contained a median of 3 million CD34+/kg

The addition of Campath to minimally immunosuppressive conditioning regimens (see boxes) may greatly improve this aspect of transplant-related morbidity and mortality and it is hoped that these combinations may reduce TRM to the levels seen in autologous transplantation. This has been observed in a study where Campath-1G was added to the conditioning regimen, BEAM (BCNU, etoposide, cytarabine and melphalan)[80], more commonly used to precede autologous transplantation. In these 12 lymphoma patients, two with CLL, Campath-BEAM produced high remission rates (75%) and a notably low incidence of GVHD. While follow-up is too short to draw conclusions about relapse rates, 75% survive and 67% remain event-free at a median of 1 year post-transplant. These results compare well with the transplant-mortality seen after autologous transplantation.

Non-myeloablative regimen plus Campath

Allografts (Kottaridis *et al.* 2000[81])

In vivo conditioning based on fludarabine:

- Campath-1H 20 mg/day iv (days –8 to –4)
- Fludarabine 30 mg/m^2 (days –7 to –3)
- Melphalan 140 mg/m^2 (day –2)
- Cyclosporine was started on day –1 as GVHD prophylaxis.

In vitro grafts:

- Sibling PBSC donors had been G-CSF mobilized days –4 to 0,
- PBSC grafts contained a median of 7 million CD34+/kg
- BM grafts contained a median of 3 million CD34+/kg

Additionally, Campath-1H has been used as an addition to non-myeloablative conditioning with fludarabine and melphalan in 44 patients with high-risk leukemia/lymphoma, 18 of whom had failed autologous transplantation[81]. Engraftment rates were high (95%) and GVHD was limited, with no cases of grade III or IV disease, although one patient developed Grade IV GVHD after DLI to treat disease relapse. Estimated probability of overall survival at 2 years was 75%, and of non-relapse mortality was 11%. At a median follow-up of 9 months, 33 patients remain alive and in complete remission or with no evidence of progression. Response and freedom from relapse were greater in patients with lymphoma (HD, NHL, or CLL) compared with those with myeloid leukemias.

Conclusions

Early results show that Campath-1H can be used as a therapeutic regimen and/or as conditioning in B-CLL, allowing patients to progress to either autologous or to allogeneic transplantation, with the elimination of residual disease in some cases. As yet, few patients have proceeded to allogeneic transplant after treatment with Campath-1H. It seems likely that advances in this field, with decreased toxicity due to non-myeloablative pre-conditioning, in prevention of GVHD, in GVHD treatment using donor lymphocyte infusions, and in improvements in stem cell yields, will see this number increase in the future, so improving the chances of remission in patients who retain residual malignant cells at transplant.

Already, a small number of heavily pre-treated B-CLL patients have achieved molecular remissions after Campath-1H therapy and attained durable remission after autologous transplantation. This raises the possibility that, by using Campath-1H as non-myeloablative therapy following by transplantation at an earlier stage of the disease, the chances of a cure may be substantially increased.

Reference List

1. Grigg A, Bardy P, Byron K, Seymour JF, Szer J. Fludarabine-based non-myeloablative chemotherapy followed by infusion of HLA-identical stem cells for relapsed leukaemia and lymphoma. *Bone Marrow Transplant.* 1999;23:107–110

2. Lossos IS, Paltiel O, Polliack A. Salvage chemotherapy using a combination of fludarabine and cyclophosphamide for refractory or relapsing indolent and aggressive non-Hodgkin's lymphomas. *Leuk Lymphoma.* 1999;33:155–160

3. Sala R, Mauro FR, Bellucci R, De Propris MS, Cordone I, Lisci A, Foa R, de Fabritiis P. Evaluation of marrow and blood haemopoietic progenitors in chronic lymphocytic leukaemia before and after chemotherapy. *Eur J Haematol.* 1998;61:14–20

4. Autologous transplantation with peripheral blood stem cells in chronic lymphocytic leukemia. A phase III, randomized, multicenter study. GIMEMA. Gruppo Italiano per le Malattie Ematologiche dell'Adulto. GITMO-Gruppo Italiano Trapianto di Midollo Osseo. *Hematol Cell Ther.* 1999;41:117–125

5. Lemoli RM, Visani G, Leopardi G, Motta MR, Rizzi S, Testoni N, Curti A, Tura S. Autologous transplantation of chemotherapy-purged PBSC collections from high-risk leukemia patients: a pilot study. *Bone Marrow Transplant.* 1999;23:235–241

6. Dreger P, Viehmann K, Steinmann J, Eckstein V, Muller-Ruchholtz W, Loffler H, Schmitz N. G-CSF-mobilized peripheral blood progenitor cells for allogeneic transplantation: comparison of T cell depletion strategies using different CD34+ selection systems or CAMPATH-1. *Exp Hematol.* 1995;23:147–154

7. Wiesneth M, Schreiner T, Bunjes D, Bischof C, Erne E, Maccari B, Kubanek B. Comparison of T-cell-depleted BMT and PBPCT with respect to chimerism, graft rejection, and leukemic relapse. *J Hematother.* 1999;8:269–274

8. Mavroudis D, Read E, Cottler-Fox M, Couriel D, Molldrem J, Carter C, Yu M, Dunbar C, Barrett J. CD34+ cell dose predicts survival, posttransplant morbidity, and rate of hematologic recovery after allogeneic marrow transplants for hematologic malignancies. *Blood.* 1996; 88:3223–3229

9. Majolino I, Cavallaro AM, Scime R. Peripheral blood stem cells for allogeneic transplantation. *Bone Marrow Transplant.* 1996;18 Suppl 2:171–174

10. Cornelissen JJ, Fibbe WE, Schattenberg AV, Petersen EJ, Willemze R, de Witte TJ, Lowenberg B, Verdonck LF, vd Biezen A, Brand R. A retrospective Dutch study comparing T cell-depleted allogeneic blood stem cell transplantation vs T cell-depleted allogeneic bone marrow transplantation. *Bone Marrow Transplant.* 1998;21 Suppl 3:S66–S70

11. Dreger P, Schmitz N. The role of stem cell transplantation in the treatment of chronic lymphocytic leukemia. *Leukemia.* 1997;11 Suppl 2:S42–S45

12. Stewart DA, Guo D, Gluck S, Morris D, Chaudhry A, Klassen J, Luider J, Auer I, Brown C, Russell JA. Low CD34+ cell dose is adversely associated with relapse-free (RFS) and overall survival (OAS) following autologous blood stem cell transplantation (ASCT). IBMTR/ABMTR. Anaheim, California; 2000:17, abstract 50

13. Reisner Y, Bachar-Lustig E, Li HW, Aversa F, Velardi A, Martelli MF. The role of megadose CD34+ progenitor cells in the treatment of leukemia patients without a matched donor and in tolerance induction for organ transplantation. *Ann N Y Acad Sci.* 1999;872:336–350

14. Rachamim N, Gan J, Segall H, Krauthgamer R, Marcus H, Berrebi A, Martelli M, Reisner Y. Tolerance induction by megadose hematopoietic transplants: donor-type human CD34 stem cells induce potent specific reduction of host anti-donor cytotoxic T lymphocyte precursors in mixed lymphocyte culture. *Transplantation.* 1998;65:1386–1393

15. Dreger P, Viehmann K, von Neuhoff N, Glaubitz T, Petzoldt O, Glass B, Uharek L, Rautenberg P, Suttorp M, Mills B, Mitsky P, Schmitz N. Autografting of highly purified peripheral blood progenitor cells following myeloablative therapy in patients with lymphoma: a prospective study of the long-term effects on tumor eradication, reconstitution of hematopoiesis and immune recovery. *Bone Marrow Transplant.* 1999;24:153–161

16. Alyea EP, Soiffer RJ, Canning C, Neuberg D, Schlossman R, Pickett C, Collins H, Wang Y, Anderson KC, Ritz J. Toxicity and efficacy of defined doses of CD4(+) donor lymphocytes for treatment of relapse after allogeneic bone marrow transplant. *Blood.* 1998;91:3671–3680

17. Glass B, Uharek L, Hartung G, Zeis M, Steinmann J, Dreger P, Kronke M, Schmitz N. Immunotherapeutic aspects of allogeneic peripheral progenitor cells. *Bone Marrow Transplant.* 1998;21 Suppl 3:S3–8

18. Soiffer RJ, Freedman AS, Neuberg D, Fisher DC, Alyea EP, Gribben J, Schlossman RL, Bartlett-Pandite L, Kuhlman C, Murray C, Freeman A, Mauch P, Anderson KC, Nadler LM, Ritz J. CD6+ T cell-depleted allogeneic bone marrow transplantation for non-Hodgkin's lymphoma. *Bone Marrow Transplant.* 1998;21:1177–1181

19. Gallardo D, Garcia-Lopez J, Sureda A, Canals C, Ferra C, Cancelas JA, Berlanga JJ, Brunet S, Boque C, Picon M, Torrico C, Amill B, Martino R, Martinez C, Martin-Henao G, Domingo-Albos A, Granena A. Low-dose donor CD8+ cells in the CD4-depleted graft prevent allogeneic marrow graft rejection and severe graft-versus-host disease for chronic myeloid leukemia patients in first chronic phase. *Bone Marrow Transplant.* 1997;20:945–952

20. Jansen J, Hanks S, Akard LP, Thompson JM, Burns S, Chang Q, English D, Garrett P. Immunomagnetic CD4+ and CD8+ cell depletion for patients at high risk for severe acute GVHD. *Bone Marrow Transplant.* 1996;17:377–382

21. Murphy WJ, Longo DL. The potential role of NK cells in the separation of graft-versus-tumor effects from graft-versus-host disease after allogeneic bone marrow transplantation. *Immunol Rev.* 1997;157:167–176

22. Gandy KL, Domen J, Aguila H, Weissman IL. CD8+TCR+ and CD8+TCR- cells in whole bone marrow facilitate the engraftment of hematopoietic stem cells across allogeneic barriers. *Immunity.* 1999;11:579–590

23. Vourka-Karussis U, Ackerstein A, Pugatsch T, Slavin S. Allogeneic cell-mediated immunotherapy for eradication of minimal residual disease: comparison of T-cell and IL-2 activated killer (LAK) cell-mediated adoptive immunotherapy in murine models. *Exp Hematol.* 1999;27:461–469

24. Pelot MR, Pearson DA, Swenson K, Zhao G, Sachs J, Yang YG, Sykes M. Lymphohematopoietic graft-vs.-host reactions can be induced without graft-vs.-host disease in murine mixed chimeras established with a cyclophosphamide-based nonmyeloablative conditioning regimen. *Biol Blood Marrow Transplant.* 1999;5:133–143

25. Siegert W, Beyer J, Kingreen D, Blasczyk R, Baurmann H, Schwella N, Schleicher J, Kirsch A, Huhn D. Treatment of relapse after allogeneic bone marrow transplantation with unmanipulated G-CSF-mobilized peripheral blood stem cell preparation. *Bone Marrow Transplant.* 1998;22:579–583

26. Drobyski WR, Endean DJ, Klein JP, Hessner MJ. Detection of BCR/ABL RNA transcripts using the polymerase chain reaction is highly predictive for relapse in patients transplanted with unrelated marrow grafts for chronic myelogenous leukaemia. *Br J Haematol.* 1997; 98:458–466

27. Wu CJ, Yang XF, McLaughlin S, Neuberg D, Canning C, Stein B, Alyea EP, Soiffer RJ, Dranoff G, Ritz J. Detection of a potent humoral response associated with immune-induced remission of chronic myelogenous leukemia. *J Clin Invest.* 2000;106:705–714

28. Ibisch C, Gallot G, Vivien R, Diez E, Jotereau F, Garand R, Vie H. Recognition of leukemic blasts by HLA-DPB1-specific cytotoxic T cell clones: a perspective for adjuvant immunotherapy post-bone marrow transplantation. *Bone Marrow Transplant.* 1999;23: 1153–1159

29. Khouri IF, Keating M, Korbling M, Przepiorka D, Anderlini P, O'Brien S, Giralt S, Ippoliti C, von Wolff B, Gajewski J, Donato M, Claxton D, Ueno N, Andersson B, Gee A, Champlin R. Transplant-lite: induction of graft-versus-malignancy using fludarabine-based nonablative chemotherapy and allogeneic blood progenitor-cell transplantation as treatment for lymphoid malignancies. *J Clin Oncol.* 1998;16:2817–2824

30. Mehta J, Powles R, Singhal S, Iveson T, Treleaven J, Catovsky D. Clinical and hematologic response of chronic lymphocytic and prolymphocytic leukemia persisting after allogeneic bone marrow transplantation with the onset of acute graft-versus-host disease: possible role of graft-versus-leukemia. *Bone Marrow Transplant.* 1996;17:371–375

31. Montagna D, Yvon E, Calcaterra V, Comoli P, Locatelli F, Maccario R, Fisher A, Cavazzana-Calvo M. Depletion of alloreactive T cells by a specific anti-interleukin-2 receptor p55 chain immunotoxin does not impair *in vitro* antileukemia and antiviral activity. *Blood.* 1999; 93:3550–3557

32. Neudorf SM, Rybka W, Ball E, Blatt J, Bloom E, Corey S, deMagalhaes-Silverman M, Koehler M, Lister J, Mierski J, Mirro J, Pincus S, Wilson J, Wollman M, Donnenberg AD. The use of counterflow centrifugal elutriation for the depletion of T cells from unrelated donor bone marrow. *J Hematother.* 1997;6:351–359

33. Frame JN, Collins NH, Cartagena T, Waldmann H, O'Reilly RJ, Dupont B, Kernan NA. T cell depletion of human bone marrow. Comparison of Campath-1 plus complement, anti-T cell ricin A chain immunotoxin, and soybean agglutinin alone or in combination with sheep erythrocytes or immunomagnetic beads. *Transplantation.* 1989;47:984–988

34. Jeong DC, Han CW, Jin JY, Kim DS, Choi IB, Kim WI, Kim HK, Kim CC, Lee BC, Imamura M, Noga SJ. Effectiveness of rotor off fraction in allogeneic murine bone marrow transplantation with complete disparity of major histocompatibility. *Exp Hematol.* 1999;27:1219–1225

35. Schaap N, Schattenberg A, Bar B, Preijers F, Geurts van Kessel A, van der Maazen R, de Boo T, de Witte T. Outcome of transplantation for standard-risk leukaemia with grafts depleted of lymphocytes after conditioning with an intensified regimen. *Br J Haematol.* 1997;98:750–759

36. O'Donnell PV, Jones RJ, Vogelsang GB, Seber A, Ambinder RF, Flinn I, Miller C, Marcellus DC, Griffin C, Abrams R, Braine HG, Grever M, Hess AD, Piantadosi S, Noga SJ. CD34+ stem cell augmentation of elutriated allogeneic bone marrow grafts: results of a phase II clinical trial of engraftment and graft-versus-host disease prophylaxis in high-risk hematologic malignancies. *Bone Marrow Transplant.* 1998;22:947–955

37. Noga SJ, Seber A, Davis JM, Berenson RJ, Vogelsang GB, Braine HG, Hess AD, Marcellus D, Miller CA, Sharkis SJ, Goodman SN, Santos GW, Jones RJ. CD34 augmentation improves allogeneic T cell-depleted bone marrow engraftment. *J Hematother.* 1998;7:151–157

38. Granena A, Castellsague X, Badell I, Ferra C, Ortega J, Brunet S, Punti C, Sureda A, Picon M, Valls A, Rutllant M, Garcia J. Autologous bone marrow transplantation for high risk acute lymphoblastic leukemia: clinical relevance of ex vivo bone marrow purging with monoclonal antibodies and complement. *Bone Marrow Transplant.* 1999;24:621 627

39. Hale G, Waldmann H. Recent results using CAMPATH-1 antibodies to control GVHD and graft rejection. *Bone Marrow Transplant.* 1996;17:305–308

40. Cobbold SP, Hale G, Clark MR, Waldmann H. Purging in auto- and allografts: monoclonal antibodies which use human complement and other natural effector mechanisms. *Prog Clin Biol Res.* 1990;333:139–134

41. Hale G, Waldmann H. CAMPATH-1 monoclonal antibodies in bone marrow transplantation. *J Hematother.* 1994;3:15–31

42. Hale G, Zhang MJ, Bunjes D, Prentice HG, Spence D, Horowitz MM, Barrett AJ, Waldmann H. Improving the outcome of bone marrow transplantation by using CD52 monoclonal antibodies to prevent graft-versus-host disease and graft rejection. *Blood.* 1998;92:4581–4590

43. Jacobs P, Wood L, Fullard L, Waldmann H, Hale G. T cell depletion by exposure to Campath-1G *in vitro* prevents graft-versus-host disease. *Bone Marrow Transplant.* 1994;13:763–769

44. Hamblin M, Marsh JC, Lawler M, McCann SR, Wickham N, Dunlop L, Ball S, Davies EG, Hale G, Waldmann H, Gordon-Smith EC. Campath-1G *in vivo* confers a low incidence of graft-versus-host disease associated with a high incidence of mixed chimaerism after bone marrow transplantation for severe aplastic anaemia using HLA-identical sibling donors. *Bone Marrow Transplant.* 1996;17:819–824

45. Clarke E, Potter MN, Oakhill A, Cornish JM, Steward CG, Pamphilon DH. A laboratory comparison of T cell depletion by CD34+ cell immunoaffinity selection and *in vitro* Campath-1M treatment: clinical implications for bone marrow transplantation and donor leukocyte therapy. *Bone Marrow Transplant.* 1997;20:599–605

46. Dao MA, Nolta JA. CD34: To select or not to select? That is the question. *Leukemia.* 2000;14:773–776

47. Osawa M, Hanada K, Hamada H, Nakauchi H. Long-term lymphohematopoietic reconstitution by a single CD34-low/negative hematopoietic stem cell. *Science.* 1996; 273:242–245

48. Bhatia M, Bonnet D, Murdoch B, Gan OI, Dick JE. A newly discovered class of human hematopoietic cells with SCID-repopulating activity. *Nat Med.* 1998;4:1038–1045

49. Goodell MA, Rosenzweig M, Kim H, Marks DF, DeMaria M, Paradis G, Grupp SA, Sieff CA, Mulligan RC, Johnson RP. Dye efflux studies suggest that hematopoietic stem cells expressing low or undetectable levels of CD34 antigen exist in multiple species. *Nat Med.* 1997; 3:1337–1345

50. Sato T, Laver JH, Ogawa M. Reversible expression of CD34 by murine hematopoietic stem cells. *Blood.* 1999;94:2548–2554

51. Nakamura Y, Ando K, Chargui J, Kawada H, Sato T, Tsuji T, Hotta T, Kato S. Ex vivo generation of CD34(+) cells from CD34(-) hematopoietic cells. *Blood.* 1999;94:4053–4059

52. Zanjani ED, Almeida-Porada G, Livingston AG, Flake AW, Ogawa M. Human bone marrow CD34- cells engraft *in vivo* and undergo multilineage expression that includes giving rise to CD34+ cells. *Exp Hematol.* 1998;26:353–360

53. Zanjani ED, Almeida-Porada G, Livingston AG, Porada CD, Ogawa M. Engraftment and multilineage expression of human bone marrow CD34- cells *in vivo*. *Ann N Y Acad Sci.* 1999;872:220–222

54. Curtis RE, Travis LB, Rowlings PA, Socie G, Kingma DW, Banks PM, Jaffe ES, Sale GE, Horowitz MM, Witherspoon RP, Shriner DA, Weisdorf DJ, Kolb HJ, Sullivan KM, Sobocinski KA, Gale RP, Hoover RN, Fraumeni JFJ, Deeg HJ. Risk of lymphoproliferative disorders after bone marrow transplantation: a multi-institutional study. *Blood.* 1999;94:2208–2216

55. Micallef IN, Chhanabhai M, Gascoyne RD, Shepherd JD, Fung HC, Nantel SH, Toze CL, Klingemann HG, Sutherland HJ, Hogge DE, Nevill TJ, Le A, Barnett MJ. Lymphoproliferative disorders following allogeneic bone marrow transplantation: the Vancouver experience. *Bone Marrow Transplant.* 1998;22:981–987

56. Hale G, Waldmann H. Risks of developing Epstein-Barr virus-related lymphoproliferative disorders after T-cell-depleted marrow transplants. CAMPATH Users. *Blood.* 1998;91:3079–3083

57. Apperley JF, Mauro FR, Goldman JM, Gregory W, Arthur CK, Hows J, Arcese W, Papa G, Mandelli F, Wardle D, *et al.* Bone marrow transplantation for chronic myeloid leukaemia in first chronic phase: importance of a graft-versus-leukaemia effect [published erratum appears in *Br J Haematol* 1988 Oct;70(2):261]. *Br J Haematol.* 1988;69:239–245

58. Davison GM, Novitzky N, Kline A, Thomas V, Abrahams L, Hale G, Waldmann H. Immune reconstitution after allogeneic bone marrow transplantation depleted of T cells. *Transplantation.* 2000;69:1341–1347

59. Flinn IW, Vogelsang, G. Bone marrow transplantation for chronic lymphocytic leukemia. *Semin Oncol.* 1998;25:60–64

60. Rabinowe SN, Soiffer RJ, Gribben JG, Daley H, Freedman AS, Daley J, Pesek K, Neuberg D, Pinkus G, Leavitt PR, *et al.* Autologous and allogeneic bone marrow transplantation for poor prognosis patients with B-cell chronic lymphocytic leukemia. *Blood.* 1993;82:1366–1376

61. Khouri IF, Keating MJ, Vriesendorp HM, Reading CL, Przepiorka D, Huh YO, Andersson BS, van Besien KW, Mehra RC, Giralt SA, *et al.* Autologous and allogeneic bone marrow transplantation for chronic lymphocytic leukemia: preliminary results. *J Clin Oncol.* 1994;12:748–758

62. Dreger P, von Neuhoff N, Kuse R, Sonnen R, Glass B, Uharek L, Schoch R, Loffler H, Schmitz N. Early stem cell transplantation for chronic lymphocytic leukaemia: a chance for cure? *Br J Cancer.* 1998;77:2291–2297

63. Jindra P, Koza V, Fiser J, Vozobulova V, Svojgrova M. Autologous CD34+ cells transplantation after FAMP treatment in a patient with CLL and persisting AIHA: complete remission of lymphoma with control of autoimmune complications. *Bone Marrow Transplant.* 1999; 24:215–217

64. Itala M, Pelliniemi TT, Rajamaki A, Remes K. Autologous blood cell transplantation in B-CLL: response to chemotherapy prior to mobilization predicts the stem cell yield. *Bone Marrow Transplant.* 1997;19:647–651

65. Scime R, Indovina A, Santoro A, Musso M, Olivieri A, Tringali S, Crescimanno A, Montanari M, Felice R, Catania P, Mariani G, Leoni P, Majolino I. PBSC mobilization, collection and positive selection in patients with chronic lymphocytic leukemia. *Bone Marrow Transplant.* 1998; 22:1159–1165

66. Schey SA, Ahsan G., Jones, R. Dose intensification and molecular responses in patients with chronic lymphocytic leukemia: a phase II single center study. *Bone Marrow Transplant.* 1999; 24:989–993

67. Dyer MJ, Kelsey SM, Mackay HJ, Emmett E, Thornton P, Hale G, Waldmann H, Newland AC, Catovsky D. *In vivo* 'purging' of residual disease in CLL with Campath-1H. *Br J Haematol.* 1997;97:669–672

68. Kennedy SM, Rawstron AC, Evans P, English A, Haynes AP, Russell NH, Byrne B, Hale G, Morgan GJ, Hillmen P. Campath-IH Therapy in 29 patients with refractory CLL: 'true' complete remission is an attainable goal. *Blood.* 1999;94:603a (abstract 2683)

69. Montserrat E, Esteve J, Schmitz N, Dreger P, Meloni G, Catovsky D, Dearden C, Scime R, Suttton L, Kimby E, Desablens B, Pavletic S, Coiffier B, Juliusson G, Besalduch J, del Potro E, Cabellero D, Michallet M. The International Project on CLL/Transplants. Autologous stem cell transplantation (ASCT) for chronic lymphocytic leukemia (CLL): Results in 107 patients. *Blood.* 1999;94:397a (abstract 1758)

70. Bandini G, Michallet M, Rosti G, Tura S. Bone marrow transplantation for chronic lymphocytic leukemia. *Bone Marrow Transplant.* 1991;7:251–253

71. Michallet M, Archimbaud E, Bandini G, Rowlings PA, Deeg HJ, Gahrton G, Montserrat E, Rozman C, Gratwohl A, Gale RP. HLA-identical sibling bone marrow transplantation in younger patients with chronic lymphocytic leukemia. European Group for Blood and Marrow Transplantation and the International Bone Marrow Transplant Registry. *Ann Intern Med.* 1996;124:311–315

72. Toze CL, Shepherd JD, Connors JM, Voss NJ, Gascoyne RD, Hogge DE, Klingemann HG, Nantel SH, Nevill TJ, Phillips GL, Reece DE, Sutherland HJ, Conneally EA, Barnett MJ. Allografting for indolent lymphoid neoplasms. *Ann Oncol.* 2000;11 Suppl 1:59–61

73. Provan D, Bartlett-Pandite L, Zwicky C, Neuberg D, Maddocks A, Corradini P, Soiffer R, Ritz J, Nadler LM, Gribben JG. Eradication of polymerase chain reaction-detectable chronic lymphocytic leukemia cells is associated with improved outcome after bone marrow transplantation. *Blood.* 1996;88:2228–2235

74. Mehta J, Powles R, Singhal S, Matthey F, Hamblin M, Middleton G, Prendiville J, Glynne P, Zomas A, Treleaven J, Catovsky D. T cell-depleted allogeneic bone marrow transplantation from a partially HLA-mismatched unrelated donor for progressive chronic lymphocytic leukemia and fludarabine-induced bone marrow failure. *Bone Marrow Transplant.* 1996; 17:881–883

75. Mehta J, Powles R, Kulkarni S, Treleaven J, Singhal S. Induction of graft-versus-host disease as immunotherapy of leukemia relapsing after allogeneic transplantation: single-center experience of 32 adult patients. *Bone Marrow Transplant.* 1997;20:129–135

76. Champlin R, Khouri I, Kornblau S, Marini F, Anderlini P, Ueno NT, Molldrem J, Giralt S. Allogeneic hematopoietic transplantation as adoptive immunotherapy. Induction of graft-versus-malignancy as primary therapy. *Hematol Oncol Clin North Am.* 1999;13:1041

77. Slavin S, Nagler A, Naparstek E, Kapelushnik Y, Aker M, Cividalli G, Varadi G, Kirschbaum M, Ackerstein A, Samuel S, Amar A, Brautbar C, Ben-Tal O, Eldor A, Or R. Nonmyeloablative stem cell transplantation and cell therapy as an alternative to conventional bone marrow transplantation with lethal cytoreduction for the treatment of malignant and nonmalignant hematologic diseases. *Blood.* 1998;91:756–763

78. Carella AM, Champlin R, Slavin S, McSweeney P, Storb R. Mini-allografts: ongoing trials in humans [editorial]. *Bone Marrow Transplant.* 2000;25:345–350

79. Nagler A, Slavin, S., Varadi, G., Naparstek., Samuel, S., Or, R. Allogeneic peripheral blood stem cell transplantation using a fludarabine-based low intensity conditioning regimen for malignant lymphoma. *Bone Marrow Transplant.* 2000;25:1021–1028

80. Cull GM, Haynes AP, Byrne JL, Carter GI, Miflin G, Rebello P, Hale G, Waldmann H, Russell NH. Preliminary experience of allogeneic stem cell transplantation for lymphoproliferative disorders using BEAM-CAMPATH conditioning: an effective regimen with low procedure-related toxicity. *Br J Haematol.* 2000;108:754–760

81. Kottaridis PD, Milligan DW, Chopra R, Chakraverty RK, Chakbarti S, Robinson S, Peggs K, Verfuath S, Pettengell R, Marsh JCW, Schey S, Mahendra P, Morgan GJ, Hale G, Waldmann H, Ruiz de Elvira MC, Williams CD, Devereux S, Linch DC, Goldstone AH, Mackinnon S. *In vivo* CAMPATH-1H prevents graft-versus-host disease following nonmyeloablative stem cell transplantation. *Blood.* 2000;96:2419–2425

Future Perspectives

Campath-1H as salvage treatment

Campath-1H offers the chance of effective therapy for refractory disease for which there is no other treatment available. It offers hope to patients who have otherwise reached the end of the line, who, without treatment, have a life expectancy measured in months.

Another potentially major effect of the availability of this treatment for refractory disease is on the decision-making process, assessing at which stage to treat B-CLL, the choice of regimens and the order of treatment. In the current situation, if a patient has become refractory to fludarabine, there is no other treatment on offer. Faced with this, fludarabine may be held 'in reserve' by physicians who are then able to offer it as a second treatment if the first option fails.

This may result in treating patients first with alkylating agent therapy, or with cladribine, then with fludarabine, despite fludarabine having proven most effective when used on untreated patients. With Campath-1H available to take the place of fludarabine as the agent of last defence, this releases the physician to more readily use fludarabine as first choice for untreated patients.

Campath-1H to complement existing therapies

As a treatment with a completely separate mechanism of action from other chemotherapies available, Campath-1H has potential to be used in combination with purine analogues, particularly fludarabine. While the combined effect of these drugs has yet to be assessed, fludarabine is already proven to be effective when used to debulk disease, and might then be followed by Campath-1H treatment to decrease residual disease. Indications of synergy of Campath-1H, with its weak anti-apoptotic effects, and potent inducers of apoptosis such as fludarabine hold the promise of strong anti-leukemic effects, and deserve further study. In addition, recent progress in the use of prophylaxis against opportunistic infections allows Campath-1H to be used with increasing safety and tolerability. Such approaches may be used as preliminaries to effective bone marrow transplantation. Campath-1H is also effective in controlling graft-versus-host disease, and so can be used with non-myeloablative conditioning prior to allogeneic transplantation in B-CLL and in other hematological malignancies.

The fact that Campath-1H can deplete both B- and T-cells may prove to be relevant to some of the unique qualities of B-CLL. Although the malignant clone arises in B-cells, the prolonged course of the disease results in long-standing aberrations in T-cell function. The cycles of remission and relapse seen in the disease when drugs are used to target the B-cell alone may be accentuated by the continued existence of dysfunctional T-cells. The use of Campath-1H to permit allogeneic transplantation for B-CLL has the advantage that both B- and T- lineages will be replaced with functioning cells.

A second factor which influences treatment choice, for refractory and for untreated patients, is the possibility that Campath-1H in combination with bone marrow transplantation can offer true remission. This casts quite a different light on prior treatment. In the situation where all treatments are palliative, the decision to stretch out the number of therapies seems reasonable despite the physical risks and mental distress of multiple and prolonged treatment regimens. Using, for instance, alkylating agents followed by cladribine followed by fludarabine, and then finally turning to Campath-1H for a final extension of remission can stretch out the duration of progressive disease through cycles of response and relapse into a period of several years. However, the situation changes dramatically if treatment using Campath-1H alone, or in combination with other therapies, can actually purge malignant cells to the extent that subsequent bone marrow transplantation can replenish the immune system with functionally normal cells. Under such circumstances, the ideal situation becomes one in which the most effective regimen is offered to patients as early as possible.

Campath-1H as emerging frontline therapy

Not only may Campath-1H ultimately find a role as a frontline treatment for B-CLL, its particular mode of action may also alter the perceptions of how early it is considered expedient to start treatment of the disease.

Historically, early treatment is considered inadvisable. This conclusion was drawn from the pioneering studies using chlorambucil alone or in combination, as initial treatment for B-CLL, comparing treatment of progressive disease to treatment of smouldering disease.

The mechanisms underlying this are threefold. The first, is that alkylating agents are potentially mutagenic and early treatment may have consequences for the later development of secondary malignancies. No equivalent work has been done to compare early and late treatment using purine analogues or other treatments which are not cell-cycle-specific. However, though it is possible that early benefits from purine analogues may be greater than for chlorambucil, they do work by a mechanism which is also potentially mutagenic, and therefore there has been no urgent motivation to reassess when treating the disease 'as early as possible' how early this can or should be.

The second, is that early, ineffective, treatment may induce development of resistant subsets of cancerous cells. Drugs with common points of metabolic intervention can provoke cross-resistance, and even in the event of no common mechanism may select for MDR (multi-drug-resistant) cells. These cells overexpress a membrane transport protein that can expel a large variety of drugs and toxins as fast as the cell can transport them inside.

The third, is that with the majority of B-CLL cells in G_0 during the indolent phase of the illness, they respond poorly to drugs which are cell cycle-specific. Many of the agents used in combination therapies, such as doxorubicin or vincristine, will therefore have relatively little effect for the dosage used.

Campath-1H has the considerable advantage that it purges in a fashion which is not mutagenic, removing this limitation to earlier treatment. This is of particular significance when offering treatment to patients who present at a relatively young age, for whom the decisions regarding treatment are exceptionally difficult. Campath-1H has no immediate theoretical disadvantages in early treatment beyond the risks inherent in immunosuppression, balanced by the advantage that patients with early disease are themselves more immunocompetent than in the later stages of the disease. Campath-1H should therefore be eminently suitable for treatment of disease as it first begins to progress. Campath-1H has become available at a time when advances have been made in using total tumor mass, measured as palpable disease or using newly available molecular markers of tumor mass, to determine the point at which disease has begun to progress and so define an appropriate moment to begin therapy. Early treatment with Campath-1H should also be seriously considered before tumor mass becomes too great or bulky node involvement develops, since Campath-1H has less effect on bulky nodal disease than on blood and bone marrow.

Other limitations to early treatment are also weakened with relation to Campath-1H; since it does not require entry to the cell, it cannot induce evasive metabolic changes, nor select for overexpression of the MDR efflux transporter. It is not cell-cycle specific. It is possible to re-treat with additional courses of Campath-1H since while CD52-negative normal lymphocytes may be selected by treatment, emergence of CD52-negative derivatives of the malignant clone seem to be very rare. The limitation of repeated treatment lies not with disease resistance but with the development of immune responses to the Campath-1H molecule. However, trials which have assayed for the presence of anti-Campath-1H antibodies during and after treatment, have found that Campath-1H almost never provokes an immune response in these patients.

Finally, Campath-1H treatment is compatible with bone marrow transplantation. Its advantage as a preliminary to autografting is that it does not interfere with the mobilization or harvesting of peripheral blood stem cells. It can provide an opportunity to enrich a stem cell population to be re-infused, with or without myeloablative conditioning by high-dose chemotherapy.

As a preliminary to allografting, it has the advantage of reducing the risk of GVHD. Further, since Campath-1H is immunosuppressive but non-myeloablative, it has much in common with other low-intensity conditioning regimens rapidly gaining acceptance because they promote rapid engraftment and reduce the risk of infection.

The emergence of Campath-1H as a safe and effective treatment for B-CLL shifts the perspective on this disease and enhances prospects of some patients to the extent that it may mark the crucial turning point when B-CLL finally becomes a curable disease.

Index

acetaminophen, use as premedication in Campath-1H trials, 71
acute leukemia, 14
administration, subcutaneous cf. intravenous, 80
adriamycin, *see* doxorubicin
age, cut-off points for in clinical trials, 71
algorithm for B-CLL treatment, 33
allografts,
  mini-BEAM-Campath, 102
  non-myeloablative regimen with Campath, 103
anemia, 11
  severe autoimmune hemolytic, 17
anti-CTLA-4, 52
anti-sense oligonucleotides, 21
antibody-dependent cellular cytotoxicity, 55
  mechanism of, 56–58
anticipation, 14
antigens, tumor-specific, 91
antiglobulin response, 51
antihistamines, use as premedication in Campath-1H trials, 71
apoptosis,
  disruption of in B-CLL, 14
  Fas-mediated, 23
  granzyme activation of, 59
  mechanisms of, 58
  mechanisms of triggering, 55
  pathways for, 22
  protection from, 20, 21
  role of growth factors in, 21
apratuzumab, 52
auto antibodies, 16
  action of, 17
autoimmune thrombocytopenia, 17
autoimmunity, 12
  Fas and, 23
  T-cell defects and, 17

β2-microglobulin,
  as a marker of early disease, 24
  as a marker of total tumor mass, 24
B-cell antigen receptor complex, 20
B-cells,
  abnormal in B-CLL, 14
  cell cycle signalling in, 19
  cross-talk, 22
  differentiation of, 15
  Fas expression on, 23
  germline rearrangements of, 15

point mutations on, 16
signal transduction in, 20
surface membrane phenotype in B-CLL, 18
B-CLL,
abnormal cells in, 14
algorithm for treatment of, 33
autoimmune phenomena in, 12
Campath-1H in refractory patients, 71–84
cell cycle signalling in, 19
cell metabolism in and treatment design, 25
chromosomal abnormality and, 12, 13
clinical course of disease, 14
diagnosis criteria, 11
ethnicity and, 14
familial risk in, 14
incidence, 11
life expectancy, 14
markers of disease progression, 24
overexpression of BCL-2 in, 20
rosette formation by lymphocytes in, 17
soluble proteins as markers of, 24
specific treatment problems of, 33
staging systems for diagnosis of, 11, 12
surface membrane phenotype of B-cells in, 18
when to treat, 14
BAK, 21
BAX, 21
BCL-2,
down-modulation of, 21
interleukin-8 levels and, 24
overexpression of, 20, 21
protein family, 20
BCL-W, 21
BCL-XL, 21
BCR-ABL tumor-specific marker, 91
BEAM therapy, 100
mini-BEAM-Campath, 102
Bexxar, 52
BFL-1, 21
Binet staging system for B-CLL, 11, 12
cf. CD23 and β2-microglobulin as survival predictor, 24
disadvantages of, 24
BL-22, 52
bone marrow infiltration and Campath-1H, 79
bone marrow transplantation,
allogeneic cf. autologous, 88
allogeneic in LGL/CLL, 101
autograft regimen, 98
autologous, 100
stem cell harvest for, 73
Campath antibodies in, 52

Campath-1H treatment prior to transplant, 87–104
engraftment, 88
CD8 and, 91
T-cells and, 91
Epstein–Barr virus-triggered lymphoproliferative disease after, 95
graft-versus-host disease, 87, 89, 90
mortality after, 97
and Campath, 102
in allogeneic, 101
non-myeloablative regimen for, 98
with Campath, 103
principles behind, 87
use in B-CLL, 96
autologous, 97
use of Campath-1H for pretransplant purging, 74

Campath antibodies,
apoptosis induction by, 58
cf. E-rosetting, 95
graft-versus-host disease reduction by, 93
humanized form, *see* Campath-1H
isotypes of, 60
stem cell recovery and, 94
technique of humanizing, 60
use as contraceptive, 55
use in bone marrow transplantation, 52
Campath-1G, graft-versus-host disease reduction by, 93
Campath-1H,
action *in vivo*, 60
trials of, 63–66
as frontline therapy, 113
bone marrow infiltration and, 79
cf. rat antibody, 62
characteristics of, 53
development of, 53
dose-escalation regimen, 65, 66, 71
dose-ranging trials, 64
durability of response, 76
early treatment with, 114
first-dose reaction against, 63
formation of humanized IgG, 61
future use as salvage treatment, 111–115
mortality reduction with in bone marrow nodal disease regression and, 78
opportunistic infections and, 64
peripheral blood stem cell harvest after, 99
phase II clinical trials of in relapsed patients, 71
premedication and, 65
prophylaxis and, 65
relapse rates, 77
repeat treatments, 77
reshaping of, 62

responses to,
in refractory patients, 75
in blood, 66
in bone marrow, 66
in bulky nodal disease, 66
side effects of, 63
first-dose reaction against, 63
lymphopenia, 63
premedications and prophylaxis for, 65
study 005, 71
administration method and response, 79, 80
residual disease, 73
response rates in, 72
toxicity in, 81
study 009, 71
response rates in, 76
study 211, 71
incidence of infections in, 82
inclusion criteria, 81
patient demographics, 82
response rates, 83
subcutaneous administration, 75
T-cell depletion by, 96
technique of humanizing, 60
to complement existing therapies, 111
use for pretransplant purging, 74
use in elderly, 71
use in refractory patients, 84
use prior to bone marrow transplantation, 87–104
Candida, 40, 82
CAP combination regimen, 36
trials of, 43
caspases, 23, 57
role in apoptosis, 59
CD4,
Campath-1H and depletion of, 63
long-term suppression of by purine analogues, 40
purine analogues and CD4+ T-cells, 17, 18
CD5,
cell surface marker expression and, 18
role in B-CLL, 15
CD8,
purine analogues and CD8+ T-cells, 17
role in engraftment, 91
CD14 as a marker of IgG serum values, 24
CD23,
as a marker of early disease, 24
as a marker of lymphocytosis and total tumor mass, 24
CD26, 19
CD27 as a marker of total tumor mass, 24

CD34,
  selection of for transplant, 94
  T-cell depletion and, 92
CD36, 19
CD38, 19
CD44, 19
  as a marker of disease progression, 24
CD52,
  characteristics of, 53
  expression of, 54
  expression on malignant cell, 55
  incidence of expression, 63
  peptide structure, 54
  recognition by Campath-1H, 53
  variant form in male reproductive tract, 55
cell cycle signalling in B-CLL, 19
cell death,
  antibody-dependent cellular cytotoxicity, 56–58
  complement-mediated cell lysis, 55–56
  lytic mechanisms, 57
  mechanisms of triggering, 55
  see also apoptosis
cell surface receptors in apoptosis, 22
chemoresistance, 33
  deletions and, 13
chemotherapy,
  resistance to,
    BCL-2 and, 21
    chromosomal abnormalities and, 13
chlorambucil, 33, 34–35
  combined with fludarabine, 43
  mode of action, 34
  response rates, 35
CHOP combination regimen, 36
  trials of, 43
chromosomal abnormality,
  benign disease and, 13
  deletions, 13
  incidence in B-CLL cells, 12, 13
  prognosis and, 13
chronic granulocytic leukemia, 14
cladribine,
  administration routes of, 38
  mode of action, 38
  opportunistic infections and, 40
  structure of, 37
  trials with, 41, 42
CLB-CD19, 52
clotrimazole, 71
CMP combination regimen, 36
combination regimens cf. fludarabine, 45

complement activation, 55
complement-mediated cell lysis, 55–56
COP combination regimen, 36
CTLA4-Ig, 52
cyclophosphamide, 35–36
  combined with fludarabine, 45
  mode of action, 35
  use in bone marrow transplantation, 97, 98
  use in combination regimens, 36
cyclosporine, use in bone marrow transplantation, 98
cytomegalovirus, 82
  reactivation of, 76
  and Campath-1H, 64

daunomycin, mode of action, 36
deletions,
  6q, 13
  11q23.1, 13
  13q14, 13
  13q14.1, 13
  17p, 13
  prognosis and, 13
deoxycoformycin, *see* pentostatin, 37
dexamethasone, use in non-Hodgkin's lymphoma, 45
disease progression, markers of, 24
DNA synthesis,
  inhibition by cladribine, 39
  inhibition by fludarabine, 39
dose-escalation regimen for Campath-1H, 65, 66
doxorubicin,
  mode of action, 36
  use in combination regimen, 36

E-rosetting,
  cf. Campath antibodies, 95
  T-cell depletion and, 93
engraftment, 87
  of peripheral blood stem cells, 97
eosinophils, role in antibody-dependent cellular cytotoxicity, 56
epirubicin, combined with fludarabine, 45
Epstein–Barr virus-triggered lymphoproliferative disease, 95
ethnicity, B-CLL and, 14

F-ara-ATP,
  modes of action, 39
  see also fludarabine
F-ara-C, RNA synthesis inhibition by, 40
famcyclovir, 71
familial risk of B-CLL, 14
Fas,
  antagonists of, 23

apoptosis mediation by, 23
expression of, 23
interactions with Fas ligand, 23
FLIP, 23
fludarabine,
active metabolite of, 39
as salvage agent, 43
as salvage therapy, 46
cf. combination therapies, 45
combined with Campath-1H, 111
combined with chlorambucil, 43
combined with cyclophosphamide, 45
combined with epirubicin, 45
current use, 81
mode of action, 39
opportunistic infections and, 40
resistance to, 46
structure of, 37
treatment of patients resistant to with Campath-1H, 64
treatment schedules for, 44
trials with, 41, 42
use in bone marrow transplantation, 98
fluorescent *in situ* hybridization, 12

germinal center, B-cells and, 16
graft-versus-host disease,
acute, 89
Campath antibodies and, 53
characteristics, 89
chronic, 89, 90
graft-versus-leukemia effect and, 90
in allogeneic bone marrow transplantation, 101
incidence, 87
links with graft-versus-leukemia effect, 92
reduction by Campath antibodies, 93
T-cell depletion control and control of, 102
graft-versus-leukemia effect, 87
graft-versus-host disease and, 90
in chronic myelocytic leukemia, 91
links with graft-versus-host disease, 92
role of T-cells in, 90
tumor-specific antigens and, 91
granulocyte colony-stimulating factor, 58
granulocyte–macrophage colony-stimulating factor, 58
granulocytopenia, purine analogues and, 40
granzymes, 57
apoptosis activation by, 59
growth factor stimuli in B-CLL, 21
growth factors, role in apoptosis, 21

Haemophilus influenzae, 12
hairy cell leukemia,
  pentostatin treatment for, 37
  secondary tumors and purine analogue treatment in, 41
hemoglobin counts in B-CLL, 12
hepatomegaly, 11
herpesvirus, 40
hLL2, 52
HulD10, 52
HuM291, 52
hybridoma technology, 51
hydroxyldaunomycin, use in combination regimen, 36
hypogammaglobulinemia, 12, 17

ibritumomab tuixetan, 52
ICAM-1, tumor spread and, 24
IgG,
  humanized Campath IgG, 62
  platelet-associated, 17
immunophenotyping, response to Campath-1H by, 74
immunosuppression,
  by mitoxantrone, 45
  by purine analogues, 40
infections, 12
  Campath-1H and, 64
  complications of and hypogammaglobulinemia, 17
  incidence of on Campath-1H, 82
  purine analogues and, 40
interferon-alpha, 36
interferon-gamma, use in late-stage B-CLL, 22
interleukin-1, thioredoxin and, 22
interleukin-2, 36
  receptor, as a marker of total tumor mass, 24
interleukin-8, BCL-2 levels and, 24
interleukin-10, use in early B-CLL, 22
irradiation, B-CLL and, 14

Legionella, 40
Listeria, 40
LMB-2, 52
lymphadenopathy, 11
lymphocytes, rosette formation by in B-CLL, 17
lymphocytosis, 11
lymphopenia, Campath-1H and, 63
lytic granules, 57

macrophages, role in antibody-dependent cellular cytotoxicity, 56
MCL-1, 21
melphalan, use in combination regimen, 36
mini-BEAM-Campath, 102

mitosis-induction protocols, 12
mitoxantrone, with fludarabine and dexamethasone in non-Hodgkin's lymphoma, 45
monoclonal antibodies,
  antiglobulin response and, 51
  characteristics of, 52
  detection in B-CLL, 12
  development of, 51–66
  production methods for, 51
multi-drug resistance trans-membrane pumps, 94
multiple sclerosis and Campath-1H, 63
mutagenesis,
  purine analogues and, 41
  secondary tumor incidence, 41

natural killer cells in antibody-dependent cellular cytotoxicity, 56
neutropenia, response to Campath-1H treatment, 73
neutrophils, role in antibody-dependent cellular cytotoxicity, 56
nodal disease,
  regression of with Campath-1H treatment, 78
  response to Campath-1H treatment, 73
non-Hodgkin's lymphoma, 20
  anti-sense oligonucleotides in, 21
  markers of disease progression, 24
mitoxantrone/fludarabine/dexamethasone for, 45
non-myeloablative regimen for bone marrow transplantation, 98
  with Campath, 103
normal autoreactive antibodies, 16

pentostatin,
  mode of action, 37
  opportunistic infections and, 40
  structure of, 37
perforin, 57
peripheral blood stem cells,
  engraftment rates with, 97
  harvest after Campath-1H, 99
platelets counts in B-CLL, 12
pneumonia, 82
point mutations in B-CLL, 16
prednisone, use in combination regimen, 36
premedication, 71, 76
  use in Campath-1H trials, 71
prognosis,
  disease progression markers, 24
  karyotypes linked with poor outcome, 13
programmed cell death, *see* apoptosis
proliferation centers, 18
prophylaxis, 71, 76
protein kinase Lck, 16
pseudo-follicles, 18

purine analogues, 36–46
metabolism of, 38
mode of action, 38
mutagenesis and, 41
secondary tumors after treatment with, 41
structure of, 37
T-cell defects after, 17
toxicity, 40
trials with, 41

Rai staging system for B-CLL, 11
disadvantages of, 24
recombinant technology, 51
refractory patients,
Campath-1H in, 71–84
response to Campath-1H, 75
relapse,
after Campath-1H, 77
cell metabolism and, 33
incidence of, 33
repeat treatments with Campath-1H after, 77
renal toxicity, side effect of purine analogues, 40
rheumatoid arthritis and Campath-1H, 63
Rituxan, 52
immune responses to, 60
rituximab, 51, 52
RNA synthesis, inhibition by fludarabine, 40
rosette formation, 17

secondary tumors after purine analogue treatment, 41
self-reactivity, 12
side effects,
antiglobulin response, 51
in repeat treatments, 79
mutagenesis, 41
of Campath-1H, 63
opportunistic infections, 40
premedications and prophylaxis for, 65
purine analogues, 40
renal toxicity, 40
tumor lysis syndrome, 40
slow proliferation, 19
soluble proteins, as disease markers, 24
spleen, response to Campath-1H treatment, 73
splenomegaly, 11
Staphylococcus spp., 12
STAT3, 16
stem cells,
Campath-1H action and, 63
harvest for autologous transplant, 73

optimum dose for engraftment, 88
recovery and Campath antibodies, 94
Streptococcus pneumoniae, 12
study 005, 71, 72
administration method and response, 79, 80
response rates in, 72
toxicity in, 81
study 009, 71
response rates in, 76
study 211, 71
incidence of infections in, 82
inclusion criteria, 81
patient demographics, 82
response rates, 83
subcutaneous administration,
local site reactions, 76
of Campath-1H, 75
response to cf. intravenous route, 80
surface membrane phenotype in B-CLL B-cells, 18
survival, predictors of, 24
systemic vasculitis, Campath-1H and, 63

T-cell activation, 16
T-cells,
defects in autoimmune complications, 17
depletion of, 92
techniques for 92–93
and graft-versus-host disease control, 102
comparison of, 95
by Campath-1H, 96
E-rosetting and, 93
engraftment and balance of, 91
Fas ligand and cell death, 23
receptors, role in engraftment, 91
role in graft-versus-leukemia effect, 90
suppression of by purine analogues, 40
therapy, *see* treatment
thioredoxin, 22
thrombocytopenia, 11
tositumab, 52
treatment,
chlorambucil, 34–35
combination regimens, 36
cyclophosphamide, 35–36
design and cell metabolism, 25
development of new, 33
resistance to drugs, 33
response rates, 35
salvage therapy, 46
see also specific treatments

timing of, 14
trials of, 41–45
trials, 41–45
CAP cf. CHOP, 43
of Campath-1H
dose escalation studies 65, 66, 71
dose-ranging trials, 64
study 005, 71–73, 79–81
study 009, 71, 76
study 211, 71, 81–84
of chlorambucil, 43
of purine analogues, 41
of treatment schedules with fludarabine, 44
trisomy 12, 13
tumor lysis syndrome, 40
tumor mass, markers of, 24
tumor necrosis factor-alpha,
role in antibody-dependent cellular cytotoxicity, 57
thioredoxin and, 22
tumor-specific antigens, graft-versus-leukemia effect and, 91

variable sequences, 16
vertical transmission, 14
VH4-34, 52
vincristine,
mode of action, 36
use in combination regimen, 36
virgin B-cells, 15

Wegener's granulomatosis (refractory), 63

Zevalin, 52